Rosemary Conley's
Amazing
Inch Loss Plan

Rosemary Conley CBE is the UK's most successful diet and fitness expert. Her diet and fitness books, videos and DVDs have consistently topped the bestseller lists with combined sales approaching nine million copies.

Rosemary has also presented more than 400 cookery programmes on television and has hosted several of her own TV series on BBC and ITV including Slim to Win with Rosemary Conley, which was first broadcast in ITV Central and Thames Valley regions in 2007, with a new series in 2008.

In 1999 Rosemary was made a Deputy Lieutenant of Leicestershire. In 2001 she was given the Freedom of the City of Leicester, and in 2004 she was awarded a CBE in the Queen's New Year Honours List for 'services to the fitness and diet industries'.

Together with her husband, Mike Rimmington, Rosemary runs five companies: Rosemary Conley Diet and Fitness Clubs, which operates an award-winning national network of almost 200 franchises running around 2000 classes weekly; Quorn House Publishing Ltd, which publishes Rosemary Conley Diet and Fitness magazine; Quorn House Media Ltd, which runs rosemaryconley.tv, an online TV channel; Rosemary Conley Licences Ltd; and Rosemary Conley Enterprises.

Rosemary has a daughter, Dawn, from her first marriage. Rosemary, Mike and Dawn are all committed Christians.

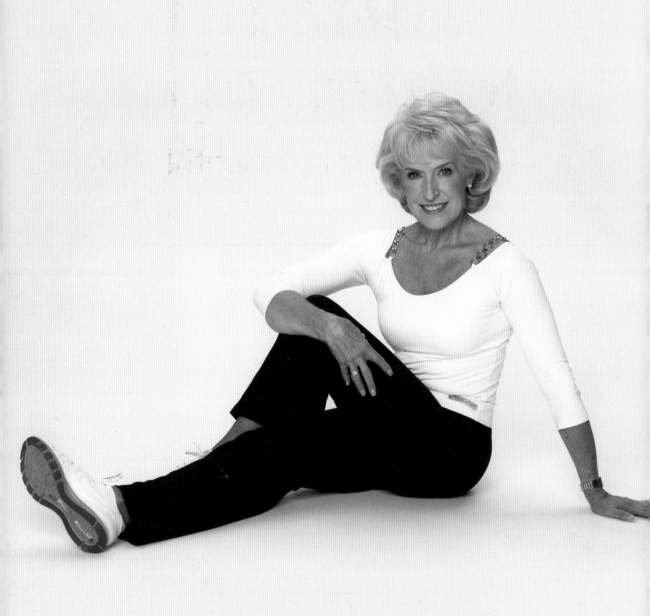

Rosemary Conley's
Amazing
Inch Loss Plan

Lose a stone in a month!

CENTURY

Published in the United Kingdom by Century in 2010

10 9 8 7 6 5 4 3 2 1

Copyright © Rosemary Conley Enterprises 2010

Century
Random House UK Limited
20 Vauxhall Bridge Road, London SW1V 2SA

Addresses for companies within The Random House Group Ltd can
be found at www.randomhouse.co.uk/offices.htm

The Random House UK Limited Reg. No. 954009

A CIP catalogue record for this book is available
from the British Library

ISBN 9781846057069

Front cover photograph by Alan Olley
Exercise photography by Alan Olley
Food photography by Clive Doyle
Edited by Jan Bowmer
Designed by Roger Walker

The Random House Group Limited supports The Forest Stewardship
Council (FSC), the leading international forest certification
organisation. All our titles that are printed on Greenpeace approved
FSC certified paper carry the FSC logo. Our paper procurement
policy can be found at www.rbooks.co.uk/environment

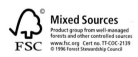

Mixed Sources
Product group from well-managed
forests and other controlled sources
www.fsc.org Cert no. TT-COC-2139
© 1996 Forest Stewardship Council
FSC

Printed and bound in Great Britain by Butler Tanner & Dennis

Also by Rosemary Conley

Rosemary Conley's Hip and Thigh Diet

Rosemary Conley's Complete Hip and Thigh Diet

Rosemary Conley's Inch Loss Plan

Rosemary Conley's Hip and Thigh Diet Cookbook
(with Patricia Bourne)

Rosemary Conley's Metabolism Booster Diet

Rosemary Conley's Whole Body Programme

Rosemary Conley's New Hip and Thigh Diet Cookbook (with
Patricia Bourne)

Shape Up for Summer

Rosemary Conley's Beach Body Plan

Rosemary Conley's Flat Stomach Plan

Be Slim! Be Fit!

Rosemary Conley's Complete Flat Stomach Plan

Rosemary Conley's New Body Plan

Rosemary Conley's New Inch Loss Plan

Rosemary Conley's Low Fat Cookbook

Rosemary Conley's Red Wine Diet

Rosemary Conley's Low Fat Cookbook Two

Rosemary Conley's Eat Yourself Slim

Rosemary Conley's Step by Step Low Fat Cookbook

Rosemary Conley's Gi Jeans Diet

Rosemary Conley's Ultimate Gi Jeans Diet

Rosemary Conley's Gi Hip and Thigh Diet

Slim to Win Diet and Cookbook

The diet in this book is based on sound healthy
eating principles. However, it is important to check
with your doctor or medical practitioner before
following any weight-reducing plan.

Contents

Acknowledgements   6

Useful information   7

How to lose weight fast!   9

Are you ready to diet?   10

Lose a stone in 28 days   14

Phase 1: 14-Day Fast Track   21

Phase 2: 14-Day 1400   110

Phase 3: Your Personal Inch Loss Plan   194
    Breakfasts   196
    Lunches   198
    Dinners   201
    Power snacks   205
    Desserts   206
    Treats   207
    Alcoholic drinks   209

Recipes: Soups   210
    Chicken and turkey   211
    Beef, lamb and pork   214
    Fish and seafood   217
    Vegetarian   218
    Desserts   222

Maintaining your new weight   226

The diet trial   227

Your personal calorie allowance   230

Index of recipes   232

Acknowledgements

I am very fortunate to work with a great team of wonderful people and I must mention some of them here.

Massive thanks must go to researcher, Sue White, who just happened to be working for me on another project, after which I was able to highjack her to help run my diet trial. It was as if it was meant to be! Sue organised all the trial dieters and supported them from beginning to end. She was also amazingly gifted at analysing the data.

Another very important member of my trial team was Bridget Key, Start-Up Manager for new franchisees at Rosemary Conley Diet and Fitness Clubs. A fully qualified diet and fitness instructor, Bridget was one of our franchisees for many years before joining our staff at head office. She supervised the technical side of our diet trial and was responsible for the health checks and weekly weighing sessions. Thank you, Bridget.

I want to make a special mention of the trial dieters, because without their determination and dedication, I would not have been able to make the 'lose a stone in a month' claim. They kindly volunteered to follow either the high protein or high carbohydrate diet in this book and, interestingly, the average weight loss was the same in both groups. Thank you all so much for being such good sports.

Thanks must go to BBC Radio Leicester presenter Tony Wadsworth, who allowed me, via his morning show, to invite volunteers for the trial. Tony, you were brilliant and I couldn't have conducted the trial without you. Thanks also to Tony's roving-reporter-wife Julie Mayer for linking up with our dieters at various intervals to see how they were progressing.

Enormous thanks must go to my dear friend and colleague, fitness expert and consultant Mary Morris, with whom I have worked for some 15 years and who has helped me to put together for this book what I believe is the most effective, progressive, exercise programme. Mary, you really are a star. Thank you!

Thanks also to Caroline Whiting, Head of Training for Rosemary Conley Diet and Fitness Clubs, for helping me with the preparatory psychological exercises that are included in this book.

I am also very grateful to Dr Susan Jebb, one of the UK's top nutritionists and an expert in weight management, for checking that the diet plan meets all the recommendations for healthy weight loss.

I have written many diet books over the years and I am delighted that so many people enjoy following them, but sometimes I need extra inspiration and for that I turn to my wonderful daughter, Dawn. Dawn is very good at keeping me on track with dieters' needs and wants, and we work together brilliantly. Thank you, as always, for your inspiration and your love.

Every diet needs good recipes so I must thank chef Dean Simpole-Clarke for his inspiration. I really don't know how you come up with such delicious creations, Dean, but you do – thankfully!

This year I have welcomed back my wonderful PA Louise Jones, who has returned to work for me now that her children are older and at school. Thank you, Lou, for all your hard work and organisational skills in helping me write and collate this marathon project, which had to be created in between the million and one other jobs I have to do. Thanks also to Anja Zeman, our executive secretary, for all your help and support.

Also, a big thank you to Susan Sandon, Emma Rose and the rest of the team at Century, for their support, encouragement and enthusiasm. Thank you also to Roger Walker, who had the unenviable task of designing this complex book and making it look appealing for the readers.

Last, but by no means least, I must say a massive thank you to Jan Bowmer, my long-suffering editor, who weaves my words into good English and ensures that the book goes to press in the right order! Bless you Jan!

Useful information

Body weight conversions

Pound (lb)	Stone (st)	Kilogram (kg)
1		0.5
2		1
3		1.4
4		1.8
5		2.3
6		2.7
7	½	3.2
8		3.6
9		4.1
10		4.5
11		5
12		5.4
13		5.9
14	1	6.3
28	2	12.7

Spoon measures

1 teaspoon = 5ml	
1 tablespoon = 15ml	

Abbreviations and symbols used

lb	pound
g	gram
kg	kilogram
st	stone
ml	millilitre
in	inch
foot	ft
mm	millimetre
cm	centimetre
kcal	calorie
tsp	teaspoon
tbsp	tablespoon
V	suitable for vegetarians
❄	suitable for home freezing
P	high protein food option

Visit www.rosemaryconley.com
for more diet and fitness advice.

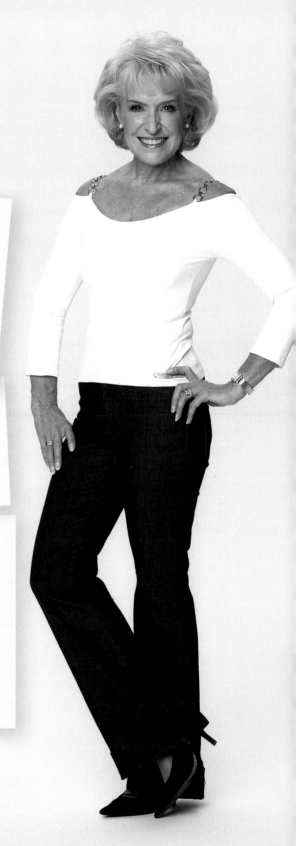

'My weight would not budge until I followed this diet. I don't feel I've been on a diet but a healthy eating plan that I plan to keep following. I feel so much better and can now wear clothes I had "grown out of"! Thank you!'
Gillian Betts (lost 1st)

'Both me and my doctor are very happy! Losing so much weight in just a month, and so easily, is amazing!'
Bill Wiltshire (lost 1st 10lb)

'I lost almost a stone in four weeks, but the biggest shock was my inch loss! I no longer suffer from heartburn or acid indigestion. I have more energy and can walk without getting out of breath. I can't believe how much food you can eat in one day!'
Jeanette Hopkins (lost 13½lb)

How to lose weight fast!

Losing weight and inches has never been easier. Why? Because this new diet has proven to be the most effective I've ever created at achieving quick weight loss and a dramatic drop in inches. In a trial involving 50 volunteers who were asked to follow the diet and take regular exercise, **the average weight loss in just four weeks was 14lb – a whole stone in a month.** It worked for them and it can work for you too!

This book not only provides all the tools you need to lose your excess weight and inches, with a 28-day programme of daily diet menus, exercises and motivation, it will also help you to get your head into the right gear before you start.

For the first time in any of my diets I have included some 'high protein' meal options in the menu plans – marked **P** – for people who like to avoid carbs or who just want to add more variety to their diet. It has been clinically proven that high-protein meals have a high satiety value, so they help us to feel fuller for longer. Of course, there are still plenty of meal choices for those who relish a good plate of pasta or a rice dish, or who like to have roast potatoes with their Sunday roast. So, whether you prefer to follow a high protein eating plan or one that gives you lots of filling, low-Gi carbohydrates, this diet has it all. It is varied and extensive and offers a vast choice of different foods to eat.

The exercise plan is designed to be quick to do and simple to follow so it can be squeezed into even the busiest of lives, while at the same time proving extremely effective. The toning exercises take only five minutes a day and there's a daily aerobic challenge where you can choose any activity that fits into your lifestyle – it could be a brisk walk in your lunch break, attending a class or working out to a fitness DVD. Do it and you'll lose weight faster.

The daily motivational tips will keep your willpower topped up, and along the journey you will learn how to speed up your weight loss, tone your muscles and turn your body into a 'fat burner' rather than a 'fat storer' so you can stay slim without ever having to 'diet' again!

Rosemary

Are you ready to diet?

You have bought this book, so I have to assume you are serious about wanting to lose weight and get fitter. But how committed are you? What has prompted your decision to shed some pounds or kilos? Self-awareness is really important and you need to identify the triggers that can trip you up and the motivators that will keep you focused on the job in hand once you embark on the diet.

Rushing into the diet without planning your campaign may not give you the results you want. Investing in a little time to assess your frame of mind and get yourself properly organised before you start could provide the key to your ultimate success.

If you find yourself saying to your friends 'I really **ought** to lose weight' or 'I **should** lose weight' and you only bought this book to show willing, you are probably being pushed into considering a weight loss plan by a third party rather than making your own decision to take action. But if you are saying '**I have decided I am going to lose weight**' and '**I am going to get fitter**' you are much more likely to succeed.

Changing the way you think about food is imperative. One of the dangers of embarking on a weight loss plan is that you can become obsessed with food. As soon as you have had one meal, you are already planning the next … and the next! Food can take on a very unhealthy importance in your mind, which almost certainly will lead to failure as you will convince yourself that you feel hungry and deprived – because you are thinking about food all the time! This needn't happen and you can retrain your brain, like I did.

Years ago when I was struggling with my own weight, I was obsessed by food – buying it, cooking it, tasting it, bingeing, dining out … In fact, food controlled my life. It was a nightmare. The more I tried to lose my unwanted weight, the more weight I gained. From originally only having a stone to lose, I ended up with almost 2½ stone to shed. Not a vast

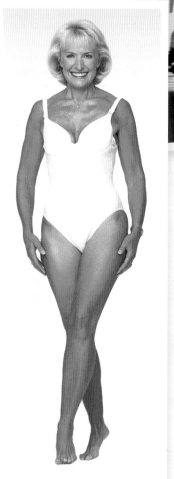

This photograph was taken in 1985 before I started eating the low-fat way.

This photograph was taken in 2000.

amount, I admit, but to someone who was only 5ft 2in tall it was significant. I hated the way I looked and my excess weight destroyed my self-esteem and affected every day of my life.

So what changed? In 1986, when I was forced on to a low-fat diet to avoid surgery for gall bladder removal, my eating habits were transformed. I had to avoid high-fat foods and found that when I cut out obvious fats like butter and cream from my diet, I lost loads of inches effortlessly. It was like a miracle. When I realised I could eat three decent-sized, healthy meals a day and keep my weight down and my body lean, I stopped seeing food as 'the enemy'. Instead, food took on a more positive role as a health-giving fuel that my body used as energy. My attitude to food changed completely and now food sits very happily in the back of my mind – rather than at the front. Consequently, I maintain my weight (within a pound or two) with very little effort.

I don't follow a 'diet' as such, but I eat low-fat foods as a matter of course. If my waistband becomes a little tight, I simply cut back for a couple of days and do a little more exercise and those extra inches quickly disappear. It works for me, so please let me help you get to this healthy point of balance too.

Most probably you will have to change the way you think about food, like I did, and you must be prepared to take action. You may need to change some behavioural patterns too. But if you have the will to do it, you can. It's all about **attitude**.

Take some time to ask yourself a few questions and have a notepad ready to jot down any thoughts or feelings. You don't have to show these to anyone else, but having them written down in black and white will help you to see more clearly how you think and feel and they will act as a useful reference point in the future. When you reach your goal weight, you'll be able to remind yourself how you felt when you started the diet and that could help you to stay slim in the long term.

Answer the following questions and jot down any thoughts and feelings:

Why do you eat the way you do?
What happened or changed in your life to cause you to gain weight?

Why do you want to lose weight?
How do you think you will feel when you have lost your excess weight?

You should find the chart on page 12 helpful as you prepare yourself for action. Why not copy it and open a folder or keep a notebook to record your progress notes? Establishing your determination to succeed is really important and you need to do everything possible to prevent lapses in your progress as you go along.

Next, it is really important to write down your goals – even those not associated with your weight or fitness. I do this all the time, as it keeps me focused and I achieve so much more that way.

Once you have reached this stage and thought about why and how badly you want to lose weight, you will have made a positive decision to do just that, as well as to get fitter and change your life for the better. You have accepted that you will have to make some changes (because if you don't you'll just get bigger) and that the likely rewards far outweigh the relatively small sacrifices you may have to make to achieve your goal.

When you have thought through your goals and the benefits you will be able to enjoy when you are slimmer, you'll find that sticking to a diet and fitness plan is relatively easy. The key is to accept responsibility and be accountable for your decisions and, ideally, find support through a class or online group. It is definitely harder to lose weight on your own.

Every week, I hear stories from members of our Rosemary Conley Diet and Fitness Clubs and our online club about how losing weight has transformed their lives – not just in a small way, but dramatically. I feel so lucky to have played a small part in helping these people achieve their new, happier and more successful lives.

Losing weight increases our self-confidence. The more confident we are, the happier we become, and the happier we are, the more we get out of life in whatever form we choose to find it. In this book I want to build your confidence and make you feel like the woman (or man) you truly want to be. I want you to be happy in your own skin and to have a sunny

Preparing to take action

List the positive aspects of following a healthy, low-fat diet and taking regular exercise (e.g. weight loss, less strain on joints, more energy, increase in confidence):

List the negative aspects of following a healthy, low-fat diet and taking regular exercise (e.g. will have to cut back on chocolate):

_____   _____

_____   _____

_____   _____

_____   _____

_____   _____

_____   _____

_____   _____

_____   _____

WHY do you want to change?
(Make a list, e.g. I want to be slim for my children; for my health; to be able to buy nice clothes)

_____

_____   _____

_____   _____

_____   _____

_____   _____

_____   _____

HOW will losing weight make you feel?
(Make a list, e.g. more attractive, less tired, more confident, fitter)

_____   _____

_____   _____

_____   _____

_____   _____

_____   _____

outlook towards your future. We only have one life, so let's make the most of it!

Developing a positive attitude

Having a positive mental attitude is crucial to your success and you may find the following guide useful in helping you to develop a more positive attitude to your weight and fitness progress. The following mnemonic was created by Caroline Whiting, Head of Training at Rosemary Conley Diet and Fitness Clubs, and she teaches it to our franchisees:

A Action required

T Take responsibility

T Turn fears into focus

I Imitate excellence

T Transform negatives into positives

U Uncover your hidden talents

D Develop yourself

E Expect the unexpected

Caroline then went a stage further and thought it would be interesting to work out where each letter of the word 'attitude' sat in the alphabet:

A = 1
T = 20
T = 20
I = 9
T = 20
U = 21
D = 4
E = 5

Add them all together and, amazingly, they come to 100! So, take these suggestions on board and enjoy 100 per cent success!

Before you start

Next, it's time to sort out your fridge and get rid of all those foods that are high in fat and that you really don't need if you're serious about losing weight. Pass them on to a slim and needy friend (or stick them in the freezer). Alternatively, just phase them out over the next week or two.

Take a look at the menu suggestions for each day of the 28-day programme and make a shopping list. The menus contain straightforward recipes and meal suggestions that require no special preparation. Your cuisine can be as simple or complicated as you choose.

Lose a stone in 28 days

The 28-day programme in this book is designed to help you through the first four weeks of your weight and inch loss journey by offering you motivation, a daily diet plan and a progressive exercise programme so that by the end of the month you will be slimmer, stronger and fitter and you will be amazed at how different you feel!

For the first two weeks of the diet, the regime is quite strict in order for you to achieve a notable weight loss in this first fortnight. This will act as a tremendous motivator, as you will see a real difference in how your clothes fit you, particularly around your waistband. The abdomen is a key target for weight loss as having a large waist size can pose a risk to your health.

In trials we have undertaken, the **average** weight loss of the trial dieters was 7.25lb in two weeks, and after four weeks they had lost an average of 14lb. So I am confident that you will lose a significant amount of weight and inches if you stick rigidly to the plan.

The diet is divided into three phases:

Phase 1: 14-Day Fast Track

Phase 2: 14-Day 1400

Phase 3: Your Personal Inch Loss Plan

The **14-Day Fast Track** diet is based on 1200 calories a day for the first two weeks. It is perfectly safe to eat this relatively low number of calories for a short, sharp kick-start of the diet. Next comes the **14-Day 1400** diet, which is slightly less strict and offers you an extra 200 calories a day – 100 to be used for a low-fat dessert or low-fat treat, plus 100 for an alcoholic drink, e.g. a 125ml glass of wine, or a high-fat treat, such as chocolate.

On Day 29, after the initial four-week diet and exercise plan, if you have more weight to lose, you can move on to the third phase: **Your Personal Inch Loss Plan**. By checking the charts on pages 230–1,

you will be able to work out your personal calorie allowance based on your weight, gender and age. This allowance will be equivalent to your basal metabolic rate (BMR), which is the number of calories that you, as an individual, burn each day just to stay alive. If you continue to diet on that number of calories, reducing the calories slightly as you lose each half stone, and you also take regular exercise, you will keep losing weight until you reach your goal.

> If at any time you want to give your weight loss a boost after a period of overindulgence, for instance after a holiday or Christmas, you can return to the **14-Day Fast Track diet**. It is not to be followed long term unless your BMR determines that 1200 calories is the correct number for your daily needs, which might be the case if you are over 60 or have a small frame, or both.

The eating plan is based on low-fat, low-Gi foods (which keep you feeling fuller for longer), with some high protein meal options (which have a high satiety value), and is combined with a daily exercise programme that will speed up your rate of weight loss, tone your muscles and boost your metabolism. There are plenty of delicious meal options for both meat-eaters and vegetarians. All the meals have been carefully selected to maximise volume and satisfaction while minimising calories and fat. Many of the recipes are ideal for entertaining and, I promise, your guests won't feel they are being presented with 'diet food'.

Why do we count calories?

Whether you follow a high protein diet or a high carb diet, calories do count. A 'calorie' is a term used to measure the energy value (fattening power) of food and drink. Different types of foods contain different amounts of calories, and foods that are high in fat contain the most. The body uses about 1200–1400 calories a day just to fuel basic bodily functions (renewing and repairing body tissue, maintaining heart and lung function, and so on). Any physical activity you do throughout the day uses extra calories on top of this basic requirement. The more you move about, the more calories you will spend, and if you undertake formal physical exercise you will increase your calorie expenditure significantly, depending on the type of activity you do, how long you do it for and at what level.

On a weight loss plan, you need to eat sufficient calories to at least meet your basic metabolic needs. If you don't, your metabolic rate will slow down to conserve energy and protect you against starvation, which is the last thing you need when trying to lose weight. You want to do everything you can to maintain your metabolic rate, and eating sufficient calories and doing extra exercise will certainly help you to achieve that.

Each day, the average woman spends in total about 1800–2200 calories (for men the figure is between 2300 and 2700) in the maintenance of basic bodily functions and in going about her daily activities. The total calorie expenditure depends on your age, weight and activity levels. If you eat fewer calories than your body uses during the day, your body has to find the extra calories to fuel its needs from somewhere else – somewhere other than food – so it draws on its fat stores, which are situated around the body, to make up the difference and the result is you lose weight. Think of your body as a bank: if its current account runs out of funds, it has to draw some cash (calories) out of its savings account (fat stores) to make up the difference.

It is really important that you consume sufficient calories to meet your basic metabolic requirements (between 1200 and 1400 for the average woman) and if you do that by eating a diet that gives you enough calories to meet that basic need, it means that every bit of activity you do – and that includes normal day-to-day moving about as well as formal exercise – will be spending fat out of your body's 'savings account' of fat and you will become slimmer. And the more exercise you do, the more fat you spend! That's why diet and exercise is so effective.

Why low fat?

Gram for gram, or ounce for ounce, fat contains twice as many calories as carbohydrate or protein, so if you eat lots of high-fat foods, you will be taking in lots of calories. Quite simply, we become fat because we eat too much fat.

Interestingly, the fat we eat is stored on our bodies to be used as an 'emergency' energy (calorie) reserve so that in times of famine we can survive for longer. Carbohydrate and protein foods are easily used by the body for fuel, but fat is 'put into storage' and is only utilised as fuel once the calories from carbohydrate and protein have been exhausted.

If you reduce the amount of fat you eat, you will be putting less fat into storage and you will get leaner. And it doesn't matter whether it is saturated or unsaturated fat – both types have the same number of calories and will be stored around your body in the same way.

When you are trying to lose weight, I recommend you aim to eat foods that have no more than five per cent fat content (that's five grams of fat per 100 grams of food), with the exception of oily fish such as salmon or mackerel once or twice a week as these contain important nutrients for heart health. If you don't eat oily fish, take a fish oil supplement instead. Some lean meats may be slightly higher than five per cent too, as are raw oats.

On my low-fat diets, I estimate the average fat intake is somewhere between 20 and 40 grams per day, whereas in the average Western diet the figure is over 100 grams. Remember, my diets are low-fat, not fat-free.

Why low Gi?

Gi stands for 'glycaemic index'. The glycaemic index was originally created to help diabetics select the most effective foods to maintain their blood glucose levels. Some foods give a sudden sugar 'rush', which causes the body's blood sugar levels to rise rapidly and then drop quickly later, and this can be dangerous for diabetics. These foods are given a 'high' Gi rating. Other foods release energy more slowly, giving a gentle and longer-lasting rise in glucose levels and then a very gradual fall, which is ideal for diabetics. These slow-energy-releasing foods have a 'low' Gi ranking.

Reading nutrition labels

Check the nutrition labels on each food product before you buy. Look at the column that gives a 100-gram breakdown for the food, then check the figure for TOTAL fat content (see sample label). All foods containing five grams or less fat per 100 grams can be eaten as part of this Amazing Inch Loss Plan, providing you stay with your daily calorie allowance.

The fat content may be broken down into polyunsaturates and saturates, but on a weight-reducing diet, this is not significant. It is the total fat content per 100 grams that is relevant in your calculations. If you follow the simple five per cent fat rule, the fat content of your food will look after itself.

Remember, keeping an eye on the calories is just as important as checking the fat content. On the nutrition label look at the TOTAL calories (kcal) per serving, alongside the ENERGY breakdown, to keep tabs on your daily intake.

NUTRITIONAL INFORMATION

typical values	amount per 100g	per 300g serving
Energy	443 kj/ 105 kcal	1329 kj/ 315 kcal
Protein	6.9g	20.7g
Carbohydrate (of which sugars)	11.2g (2.6g)	33.6g (7.8g)
FAT (of which saturates)	3.7g (1.7g)	11.1g (5.1g)

Even though there is a total of 11.1g fat in each serving, there is still only 3.7g fat per 100g (3.7%), making it a low-fat food.

As you can see, this food contains 315 calories per 300g serving. Keep this figure in mind when planning your menus.

In addition, doctors found evidence of improved heart health in diabetics who followed a low-Gi diet. So it was established that eating a low-Gi diet was good for everyone, not just diabetics. Soon there was a deluge of books published on the subject and low-Gi eating became very fashionable. Nevertheless, it is accepted by nutritionists and doctors alike that eating a diet rich in low-Gi carbohydrates is good for all of us.

For the dieter, eating a diet rich in low-Gi foods is very helpful, as the very nature of low-Gi foods is that they help keep blood sugar levels stable and keep you feeling fuller for longer, which is ideal for anyone on a reduced-calorie eating programme. And eating low Gi is easier than you think. Just make some simple low-Gi choices when shopping for carbohydrates and include these in your menus, and you will automatically be eating a low-Gi diet.

LOW-GI CHOICES

■ **Bread** Choose brown wholegrain or multigrain bread or bread made from stoneground flour. Pitta bread is also low Gi.

■ **Pasta** All pasta is low Gi. Eat it with low-fat, tomato-based sauces in preference to creamy ones when you are trying to lose weight.

■ **Rice** Basmati rice is the best choice as it has a lower Gi than most other types.

■ **Potatoes** Choose sweet potatoes in preference to old ones. Waxy new potatoes are also low Gi. Cook and eat them with their skins intact to add fibre to your diet.

■ **Breakfast cereals** Go for high-fibre cereals (like All-Bran, Bran Buds, Grape Nuts and Fruit 'n' Fibre) or cereals containing wholegrain (e.g. Shredded Wheat and Special K). Oat-based varieties (such as porridge or muesli) are usually low Gi. Watch out for 'cluster' types of cereal as these can contain a lot of extra fat and sugar.

Why exercise?

Exercise burns extra calories, which helps us to lose weight faster.

Aerobic exercise – that's any exercise which makes us breathe more deeply and take in extra oxygen – burns fat from our body's fat stores as fuel, so it should always be included in a weight-loss programme. Moreover, aerobic exercise increases our metabolic rate, not just during the activity itself but also for several hours afterwards. Each day on this programme I ask you to do some aerobic activity and once a week I ask you to do a 45–60 minute session, which could be an aerobics class or working out to a fitness DVD at home.

Toning and **strength** exercises make our muscles stronger and give us a better shape. As muscle tissue is energy-hungry, the stronger our muscles, the higher our metabolic rate and the more efficient our bodies will become at burning fat. On six days a week in this plan I ask you to do a few specific exercises that target the major muscles in the body. The toning sessions only take five minutes and they become more challenging throughout the 28 days. If you follow the programme accurately you will be amazed at how quickly you progress to the more difficult exercises that will prove even more effective at toning your muscles and giving you a great figure. They really will transform your body!

There is a real synergy between aerobic and strength exercise. During aerobic exercise, the extra oxygen that we breathe in through our lungs is transported around the body and into our muscles via the bloodstream. Muscles contain thousands of little engines called 'mitochondria' which fire up during aerobic exercise, but to do this they need fuel. So the mitochondria 'power houses' call on the fat stores around the body and, with the help of the extra oxygen from the aerobic activity, they burn that fat for fuel. The result is the fat burns in the oxygen flame, and we use up some of our stored body fat!

The stronger our muscles, the more mitochondria we grow and the more fat we can burn. That's why combining aerobics with toning and strength exercises is so effective in helping us achieve a leaner body and it also helps to keep our bones healthy and strong.

Ideally, work out aerobically five times a week for around 30 minutes and do some strength exercises on most days a week – they need only take five minutes. If you do the exercises in this book, you will change your body from being a 'fat storer' into a 'fat burner' in no time and this will help you to stay slim in the long term.

The bottom line is that exercise makes us slimmer, fitter and healthier and gives us a better figure. Just do it!

> All the classes at a Rosemary Conley Diet and Fitness Club include a 45-minute workout, which incorporates a combination of aerobic and toning exercises. For details of your nearest class visit www.rosemaryconley.com

What about alcohol?

Most people love having a drink with their friends and, indeed, some alcohol in moderation can be good for our health. I am the first to admit I love a glass of wine, so I am not about to tell you that you should give it up. 'Phew!' I hear you say. But problems arise when alcohol is drunk in excess and, for some people, it is the main cause of their weight problem.

Let's look at some facts. Alcohol contains a lot of calories that offer no nutrients. As alcohol is a toxin, the body will always process it quickly, burning it away as energy as a top priority before it processes the carbohydrate, protein and, of course, the fat that you've eaten. The consequence of this is that your half bottle of wine will have used up 250 calories of your daily allowance, and the excess calories from any food you have eaten will have been deposited as fat around your body rather than being burned away, because the calories from alcohol have jumped the queue and taken precedence.

The other factor is that alcohol weakens our willpower, so we are much more likely to say to ourselves, 'Oh, forget the diet today, I'll be good tomorrow!' Then to cap it all, when we drink a lot of alcohol we tend to fancy fatty foods! Crisps and peanuts, pizzas and curries are usual choices, with disastrous results for the dieter. If this is only a rare occurrence, that's fine, but if it happens regularly, you need to change your lifestyle if you are serious about losing weight!

Let's get started!

Step 1

Before you start this diet and fitness programme, make sure you have the appropriate food in the house and that you have discarded or donated any foods that might tempt you from the amazing benefits you are going to enjoy. Check that you have some suitable footwear for exercise and that you have told your family and friends what you are aiming to do. Enlist their support and encouragement. Tell them why you are doing this and that everyone will benefit if you lose your excess weight (you'll be much happier, which has to be of benefit to them!).

Step 2

Decide on your start day and weigh yourself first thing that morning and then again each week, at the same time of day and on the same scales. Measure yourself too, either using a tape measure or, if you have one, my Magic Measure®. This is a special tape measure that comes with a series of colour-coded, clip-on tags, some permanent and some removable, and each colour represents a different part of the body (bust, waist, hips, etc.). You clip a permanent tag on to the tape measure to register your 'start' measurements, then at your future measuring sessions you clip a removable tag in the hole at your nearest inch measurement. This will enable you to see your progress from the first day of your weight and inch loss campaign.

If you don't have a Magic Measure®, take your measurements anyway on Day 1 and write them down on a piece of paper and, when you get your Magic Measure®, you can clip your 'start' markers on your 'start' measurements on the tape accordingly. Alternatively, just make a note of your details at the back of this book or in your notebook or folder.

Step 3

Before you start the programme, take a photograph of yourself (or ask someone else to take it) wearing something unflattering. This photo is going to inspire you to stick with the programme and also give you incredible encouragement as you see your progress over the coming weeks and months. Take a new shot every four weeks and place them in your personal diet folder or notebook. You will be so glad you did when you reach your goal weight and you look back and see how far you've come. You never know, you might be selected to feature in my *Diet & Fitness* magazine – and some of you might even make it to the front cover! To be considered, you will have to write to me with full details of your weight and inch loss and any relevant stories, enclosing clear 'before' and 'after' shots and your contact information.

All the slimmers who are featured in the magazine come to our head offices at Quorn House, in Leicestershire. We go shopping to choose the clothes for the day, then return to the studio at Quorn House where each slimmer has a makeover with a professional make-up artist before being photographed by one of the UK's top photographers. To finish off the day, I interview them for Rosemaryconley.tv, our television channel on the web. It is a magical day and everyone really enjoys themselves.

We are always inspired when we meet these successful slimmers and hear their amazing stories – and next year, it could be you!

How to follow the 28-day programme

During the first two weeks of the **14-Day Fast Track** diet, you are allowed three meals a day – one breakfast, lunch and dinner – plus two power snacks, one mid-morning and one mid-afternoon. You can follow the diet menus I have suggested, or choose any breakfast, lunch or dinner in this book. In addition you should consume 450ml (¾ pint) skimmed or semi-skimmed milk, which you can take on cereals and in teas and coffees as you wish throughout the day. I ask you not to drink any alcohol during these first two weeks. Sorry – but it is only for this short period (you'll be able to enjoy a drink in Week 3) and going without for these two weeks will have a dramatic effect on your weight loss.

From Week 3, on the **14-Day 1400** diet, you can have an extra 200 calories a day (1400 in total). So, in addition to your three meals and two power snacks, you can enjoy an alcoholic drink or a high-fat treat like chocolate or crisps (max. 100 kcal) plus a low-fat pudding or treat (max. 100 kcal). If you wish, you can save up your 'treat' calories over a week (max. seven days, 700 calories) for a bigger, high-fat treat or a night out on the town! Of course, you may also choose to use these 'treat' calories for low-fat food. It's up to you.

All the meal suggestions are calorie-counted and all are interchangeable within each category, providing you swap like for like, e.g. one breakfast for another breakfast, and aim to include five portions of fruit and/or vegetables each day. The diet plan I recommend is a balanced one, but because our personal needs vary, I recommend that you take a multivitamin supplement daily to ensure you get all the vitamins you need.

If you have a set of my Portion Pots® (these are handy tools for measuring everyday foods such as breakfast cereals, rice and pasta quickly and accurately), use them to measure your portion sizes – don't guess or you may overestimate your serving sizes and end up not losing as much weight as you expect to. For readers who don't have a set I have given the equivalent metric measures.

Cook without fat and don't add any fat during your food preparation. Grill or dry-fry foods instead of frying (or use a little spray oil). When cooking vegetables, rice and pasta, add a vegetable stock cube to the cooking water for extra flavour.

Do the toning exercises and the aerobic challenge as described for the first 28 days. The toning programme is progressive, so each day the exercises become more challenging. As you proceed through the programme, if you find it difficult to complete the more advanced moves, just repeat the earlier versions of the exercises until you feel ready to progress.

Diet notes

Milk
Make sure you consume 450ml (¾ pint) skimmed or semi-skimmed milk a day for use on breakfast cereals and in teas and coffees. If you are allergic to or intolerant of cow's milk you may have soya or rice milk instead. If you don't drink much milk, you may substitute 125ml low-fat yogurt (max. 75 kcal) for 150ml (¼ pint) milk.

Bread
Choose wholegrain, multigrain or stoneground bread. In these menu plans, one slice of wholegrain bread has 100 calories.

Breakfast cereals
Choose high-fibre cereals (e.g. All-Bran, Fruit 'n' Fibre, Bran Buds and Grape Nuts) or ones containing wholegrain (such as Shredded Wheat and Special K). Oat-based varieties (e.g. porridge or muesli) are usually low Gi. Watch out for 'cluster' types of cereal as these can contain a lot of extra fat and sugar.

Fruit and vegetables
Aim to eat five portions or fruit and/or vegetables each day. A portion of fruit is one small orange, apple or pear or a regular kiwi fruit, nectarine or peach or 115g fruit such as berries or grapes. In the diet plan this is described as '1 piece fresh fruit'. Approximately 1 × 115g serving of vegetables counts as one of your 5-a-day portions. All vegetables should be cooked and served without added fat. 'Unlimited vegetables' means any vegetables except potatoes.

Salad
Salad includes all salad leaves, cress, tomatoes and raw vegetables such as cucumber, peppers, carrots, onion, mushrooms, celery and courgettes, and may be served with any low-calorie, fat-free dressing, balsamic vinegar or soy sauce. Avoid pre-packed or ready-made salads with dressing as most are high in fat.

Gravy
Make gravy with gravy powder or low-fat granules.

Oily fish
For good heart health it is important to eat two portions a week of oily fish, e.g. mackerel, salmon, sardines, herrings, even though this exceeds my five per cent fat ruling.

Drinks
Regular and fruit teas and coffee made with water are unrestricted. Use milk from your daily allowance as required. All low-calorie and diet drinks may be drunk freely. Water is also unrestricted – aim to drink 2 litres a day.

means suitable for vegetarians or vegetarian option is available.

 means suitable for freezing.

 means this is a high-protein meal choice.

Remember, all meals are interchangeable within each category, so you can swap or repeat your favourites as you wish.

Throughout this book, I occasionally mention products or services that help people to lose weight and get fitter. At Rosemary Conley, we spend a lot of time and effort to find gadgets, products and services that we genuinely believe will help you on your weight loss journey. Everything has been personally chosen by me, whether it be a pedometer, a set of Portion Pots®, my Magic Measure® or a milk jug, and nothing is offered unless I am satisfied that it is of the highest standard. If at any time our goods or services do not meet those high standards, please let me know.

Perfect portion control

Overestimating portion sizes is the biggest single reason why dieters don't lose weight as fast as they think they deserve to.

Rosemary Conley Portion Pots, which come in four different sizes and colours, offer a simple solution for measuring your servings of staple foods such as rice, pasta, cereals, baked beans, chopped foods – and even wine. Once you get into the habit of using them, you'll speed up your weight loss like a dream. To order a set, visit www.rosemaryconley.com or call 0870 050 7727. They cost just £4.99 plus p&p or get a set free when you join your local Rosemary Conley Diet and Fitness Club.

I have included the appropriate Portion Pot® colour in the diet and menu plans to help you measure your servings with greater accuracy and ease, but in case you do not yet own a set I have also given the metric weight equivalents.

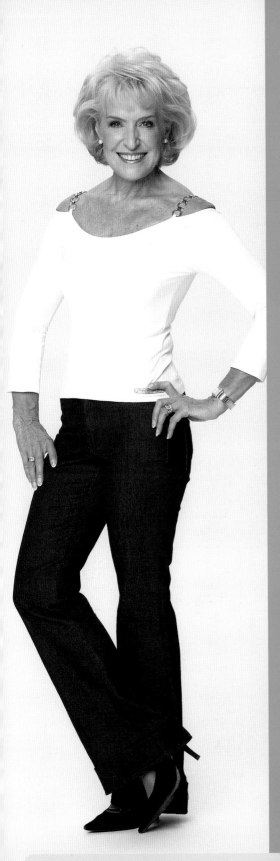

THE 28-DAY PLAN

Weeks 1 and 2
Phase 1: 14-Day Fast Track

Weeks 2 and 3
Phase 2: 14-Day 1400

Daily allowance

Throughout the diet the calories have been allocated as follows:

Breakfast	200 kcal
Mid-morning Power Snack	50 kcal
Lunch	300 kcal
Mid-afternoon Power Snack	50 kcal
Dinner	400 kcal
450ml (¾ pint) skimmed or semi-skimmed milk	200 kcal
Total (Weeks 1 and 2)	**1200 kcal**

Add-ons from Week 3

1 alcoholic drink OR high-fat treat	100 kcal
1 low-fat dessert OR low-fat treat	100 kcal
Total (Weeks 3 and 4)	**1400 kcal**

Phase 1:
Day 1

This is an exciting day! It marks the start of one of the most important journeys of your life. That might sound dramatic, but imagine how different you will look and feel in one month! As you continue on the programme you will realise that losing weight is life-changing, and you have already taken the first big step.

Have you read the first few pages of this book? If not, please do so now before you begin this programme. Otherwise it's like buying a new gadget and ignoring the instructions in your haste to get started. These pages contain vital information on how the programme works and how to maximise your progress.

I hope you enjoy today's menu. If there's a meal suggestion you don't fancy, feel free to flick through the book and find an alternative meal in the same category (e.g. swap a lunch for another lunch option) to suit your taste and your lifestyle. That's the beauty of this diet, it's so versatile.

Find a suitable time to do the exercises to fit them around your other activities. If you are really busy, it's a good idea to do them first thing, before you shower, so they don't get squeezed out of your schedule later. Exercising first thing will also strengthen your willpower throughout the rest of the day. Today's five-minute tone-up targets the waist, abdominals, backside, chest and those horrible flabby underarms! Make sure you warm up first. You can do the warm-up I have suggested or choose one from another day. All the warm-ups in this book are designed to gently stimulate your cardiovascular system and loosen the major joints before you start exercising. Alternatively, if you plan to do the exercises later in the day, you could do them after walking the dog or vacuuming your living room, as activities like this will also warm up your body.

Have you weighed and measured yourself? If not, do it now. Lastly, find an old belt and, using a marker pen, make a mark on the belt where it fits around your waist and write today's date on it too. Or consider ordering a Magic Measure® (www.rosemaryconley.com). If you join one of our classes, you'll receive one free in your membership pack.

MENU

Breakfast
■ 2 well-grilled back bacon rashers or 2 Quorn sausages, grilled, served with 1 dry-fried medium-sized egg, 3 tomatoes, halved and grilled, and 5 grilled mushrooms ✓ P

Mid-morning power snack
■ 150g strawberries ✓

Lunch
■ 1 × 400g can any soup (max. 150 kcal and 5% fat). Plus 1 Müllerlight yogurt, any flavour (max. 150 kcal)

Mid-afternoon power snack
■ 1 rice cake spread with 20g Philadelphia Extra Light soft cheese and sliced cucumber ✓

Dinner
■ Pasta Bolognese: Dry-fry 100g lean minced beef or Quorn mince in a non-stick pan, seasoning well with black pepper. Drain off the fat, add ½ chopped onion, 1 crushed garlic clove and ½ chopped red pepper and dry-fry until soft. Stir in ¼ jar Dolmio Bolognese Original Light Pasta Sauce and 1 × 200g can chopped tomatoes and simmer for 10 minutes. Serve with 1 yellow Portion Pot® (45g uncooked weight) pasta shapes, boiled with a vegetable stock cube ✓
OR
■ Black Bean Prawns (see recipe, p.217) served with 1 blue Portion Pot® (55g uncooked weight) or 1 red Portion Pot® (144g cooked weight) boiled basmati rice. Plus 1 Marks & Spencer meringue nest topped with 1 tsp 0% fat Greek yogurt and 1 tbsp raspberries

WARM-UP

March on spot with shoulder rolls

Stand tall and march on the spot for a total of 2 minutes. For every 4 steps, do a full shoulder roll, pulling shoulders forward, up, back and down.

FIVE-MINUTE TONE-UP

1 Waist trimmer ▼

(2 × 10 reps alternate sides)

Stand tall with feet slightly wider than hip width, knees slightly bent and tummy pulled in, and hold a water bottle or handweight in each hand. Keeping hips still, bend from waist to one side without leaning forward or back. Come up and repeat to other side. Keep changing sides for 10 reps (5 each side). Rest for a few seconds, then do another set.

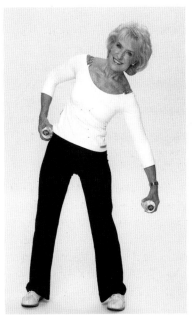

2 Underarm toner

(2 × 10 reps)

Still holding weights or water bottles, lean forward from hips, keeping your back straight, and place hands on waist with elbows pushed back Ⓐ. Now straighten elbows, pressing forearms behind you without locking elbows Ⓑ, then bring hands back to waist, and repeat. Keep shoulders down and back and head in line with spine. Do 10 reps, then rest before doing another set.

Ⓐ

Ⓑ

3 Chest shaper ▶

(2 × 8 reps)

Lie on back with knees bent, with weight or water bottle in each hand, arms bent at right angles at sides and elbows in line with shoulders Ⓐ. Now breathe in and, as you breathe out, extend arms above chest without locking elbows Ⓑ. Lower again under control and do 8 reps in total, then rest before doing another set.

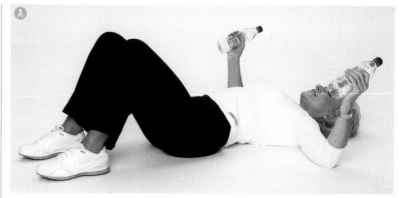

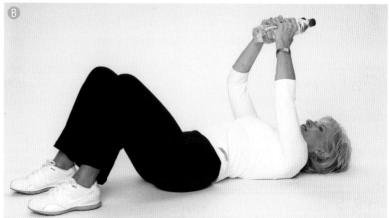

4 Bottom shaper ▶

(2 × 8 reps)

Lie on back with knees bent, feet parallel and placed close to hips Ⓐ. Slowly lift hips off floor, squeezing your bottom muscles, without arching your back Ⓑ. Keep your neck and shoulders relaxed. Lower again under control, and repeat. Do 8 reps, then rest before doing another set.

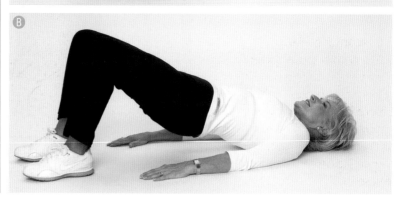

5 Tummy curl ▶

(2 × 8 reps)
Lie on back with knees bent and feet hip width apart. Place right hand behind head and left hand on top of left thigh. Breathe in and, as you breathe out, lift head and shoulders off floor, pulling your tummy in tight. Lower again slowly, keeping your tummy in. Do 8 reps, keeping your tummy in, then rest before doing another set.

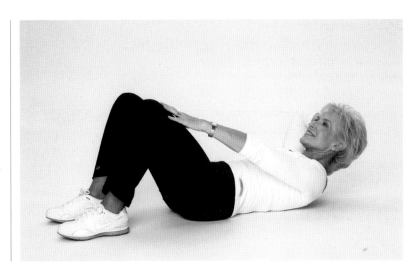

POST-WORKOUT STRETCHES

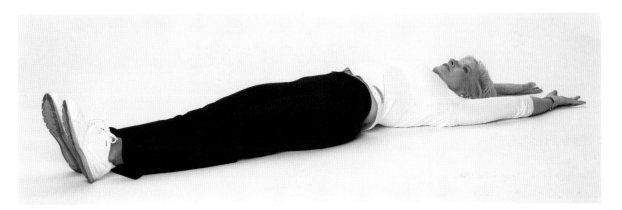

1 Tummy stretch ▲

Lie on back with legs straight and take arms overhead. Stretch arms away from legs to feel a stretch down your tummy, and hold for 10 seconds.

2 Bottom stretch ▶

Still lying on back, bend knees and place feet flat on floor. Take hold behind knees and bring them closer to your chest, to stretch the back of your hips. Keep your head on floor with neck and shoulders relaxed. Hold for 10 seconds, then release.

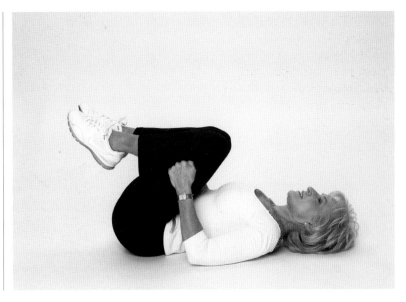

3 Underarm stretch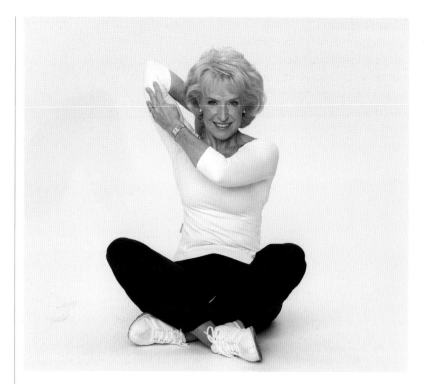

Sit upright with legs crossed and place right hand behind right shoulder. Press left hand on right underarm to push right hand further down your back. Keep your head up and look straight ahead. Hold for 10 seconds, then change arms and repeat.

4 Waist stretch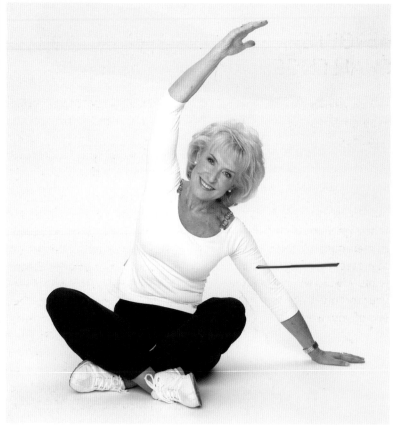

Still sitting up tall with legs crossed, lift right arm and lean over to left side, keeping both hips on floor and without leaning forward or back. Hold for 10 seconds, then change sides and repeat.

5 Chest stretch ▶

Sit upright and place both hands behind you on floor. Draw shoulders back to feel a stretch across chest, and hold for 10 seconds.

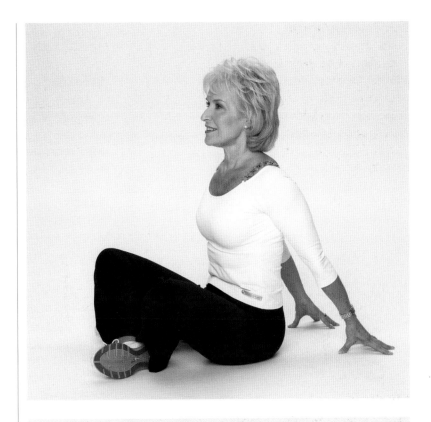

AEROBIC CHALLENGE

Go for a 20-minute walk and then do the stretches on pp.47–51 (Day 5) to finish.

Exercise tip

Make sure you wear comfortable fitness gear and always wear trainers during aerobic exercise to protect your feet, legs and joints. Always warm up before you start and then stretch at the end of your workout.

MOTIVATIONAL THOUGHT FOR THE DAY

Take a really good look at yourself in the mirror today, wearing just your underwear, so that you can face up to your body and where you are now, then confirm to yourself that this is the first day of a journey towards a new you. Say out loud that you are embarking on this weight loss plan for YOUR benefit, and no one else's.

Now I would like you to detach yourself from your reflection in the mirror and, instead of seeing yourself, think of that image as your new best friend, the one you are going to help to lose weight. Don't shy away from talking to that image in the mirror as you lose your excess weight and inches. Be encouraging and be complimentary. Look at the good features of this new friend – maybe their eyes, skin, hair, face, nails, or even their feet. It is important to get rid of any feelings of self-loathing you may have and to start respecting this person, who is totally worthy of your friendship and support. It's much easier to have respect for yourself if you see yourself as another person. From now on, stop being negative or putting yourself down – you wouldn't do that to a friend – and start complimenting yourself. Become your own best friend.

Day 2

I hope that yesterday went well and that you managed to stick to the diet and do the exercises. You probably slept better than usual as you won't have felt so bloated or lethargic and the extra exercise should have helped too. Avoid popping on the scales just yet – wait until next week when the difference will be more noticeable and you will get a more accurate result. Our weight can fluctuate from one day to another, so weekly weigh-ins are more helpful than daily ones.

If you are not normally a breakfast-eater, hopefully you managed to eat at least something before 10 a.m. People who eat breakfast tend to weigh less than those who don't, so please make the effort to get into the habit.

You will need a sturdy dining chair for today's toning exercises, which will work the waist, backside, thighs and the posture muscles. Although these exercises take only five minutes, they are really effective.

MENU

Breakfast
- 1 green Portion Pot® (50g) Special K cereal plus milk from allowance and 1 tsp sugar ✓

Mid-morning power snack
- 12 seedless grapes ✓

Lunch
- 100g cooked chicken breast (no skin), sliced, served with a large mixed salad and 1 tbsp Hellmann's Extra Light Mayonnaise **P**
OR
- 1 × 50g wholemeal pitta bread filled with 50g low-fat houmous and chopped mixed salad sprinkled with low-fat dressing of your choice ✓

Mid-afternoon power snack
- 20g low-fat cheese* (max. 5 % fat) plus 5 cherry tomatoes ✓

Dinner
- 1 × 115g (raw weight) salmon steak, steamed or microwaved, served with 80g boiled new potatoes (with skins), plus 1 yellow Portion Pot® (70g) frozen or canned peas, 100g steamed broccoli or asparagus and 1 tbsp Hellmann's Extra Light Mayonnaise
OR
- 1 low-fat veggie burger (max. 180 kcal and 5 % fat, e.g. Grassington's Vegetable Quarter Pounder or Quorn Quarter Pounder) cooked as per instructions. Serve with 115g boiled new potatoes (with skins) and a large salad tossed in low-fat dressing ✓

* Rosemary Conley mature cheese contains 5 % fat and is available by mail order via www.rosemaryconley.com

WARM-UP

Ski swings

Stand tall and lift both arms overhead. Pull tummy in and swing arms down and past your thighs as you bend your knees and hips. Keep your back straight and keep looking forward. Come up again and repeat ski swings for 1 minute.

FIVE-MINUTE TONE-UP

1 Seated side bend ▼
(2 × 10 reps alternate sides)

Sit on front third of chair seat, holding a handweight or water bottle in each hand. Pull tummy in very tight and bend to one side without dropping forward or back, then come back to centre and bend to other side. Do 10 reps (5 each side), keeping it slow and controlled, then rest before doing another set.

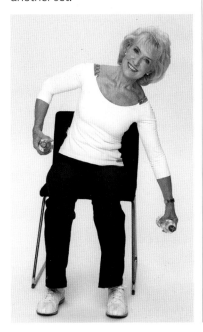

2 Posture improver
(2 × 8 reps)

Sit upright with a weight or water bottle in each hand and each arm bent at 90 degrees as if you were holding a large tray Ⓐ. Keeping elbows close to waist, pull hands further apart Ⓑ and pull shoulders down to feel shoulder blades working. Return to start position and do 8 reps slowly, then rest before doing another set.

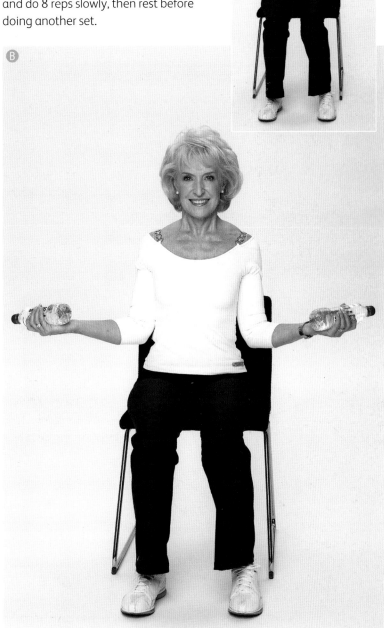

3 Stand up sit down ▼

(2 × 10 reps)

Stand tall in front of chair with feet parallel and hip width apart Ⓐ. Now bend knees and hips back towards chair seat to sit down Ⓑ and just touch the seat lightly before lifting up again. Keep lowering and lifting for 10 reps, and build up to 2 sets of 10. Keep knees hip width apart at all times and keep your back straight.

4 Standing thigh trimmer ▼

(× 16 reps alternate sides)

Stand and hold on to back of chair with feet hip width apart, body upright and tummy pulled in. Bend both knees slightly Ⓐ, then lift left leg out to side Ⓑ, keeping leg straight and foot turned in slightly. Bring leg down again, bending knees, before taking other leg out to side. Do 16 reps (8 each side).

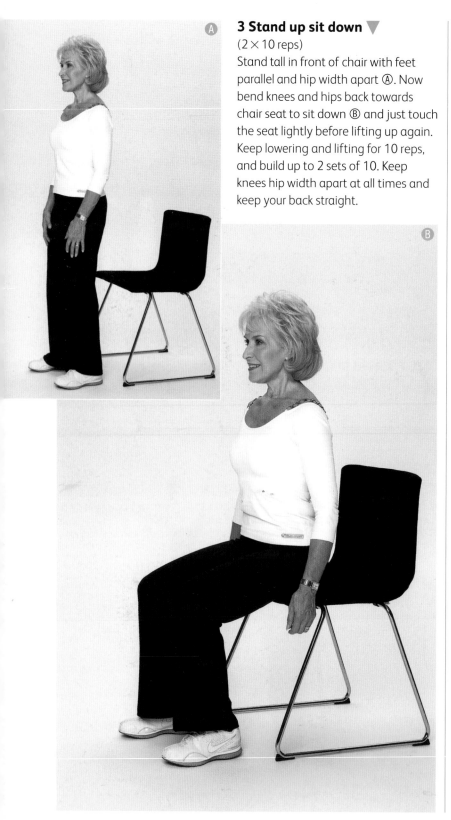

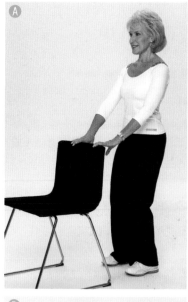

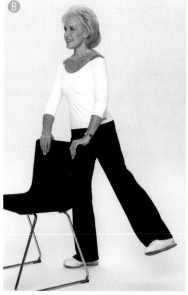

5 Bottom lifter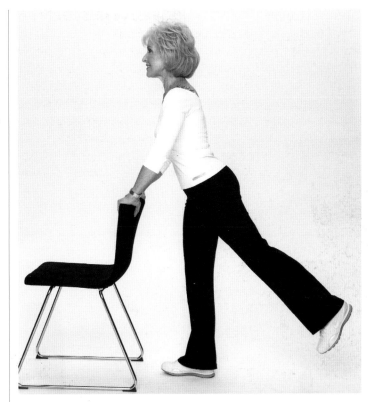
(× 16 reps alternate legs)
Still standing behind chair, lean forward slightly and pull tummy in. Keep hips facing front all the time as you lift left leg back and up, leading with heel. Bring leg down again and bend knees slightly before taking right leg back and up. Keep changing legs in a smooth and rhythmical way for 16 reps (8 each leg).

POST-WORKOUT STRETCHES

1 Upper back stretch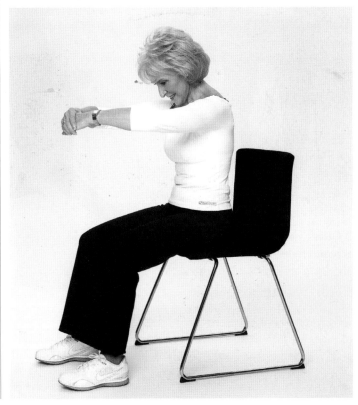
Bring both arms forward at chest height and drop head down. Press arms forward and shoulder blades back to feel a stretch across upper back. Hold for 10 seconds, then release.

2 Waist stretch ▼

Sit on front third of chair seat and lift left arm, keeping right hand on chair seat for support. Keeping both hips firmly on chair seat, bend to right without leaning forward or back, and feel a stretch down the left side. Hold for 10 seconds, then change sides and repeat.

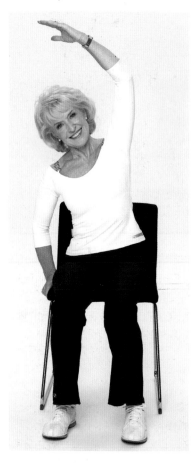

3 Outer thigh and hip stretch ▶

Bring one ankle onto opposite knee and, holding chair seat for support, let the knee drop outwards to feel a stretch in the outer thigh and hip. (If this is too difficult, just cross the legs.) Hold the stretch for 10 seconds, then change legs and repeat.

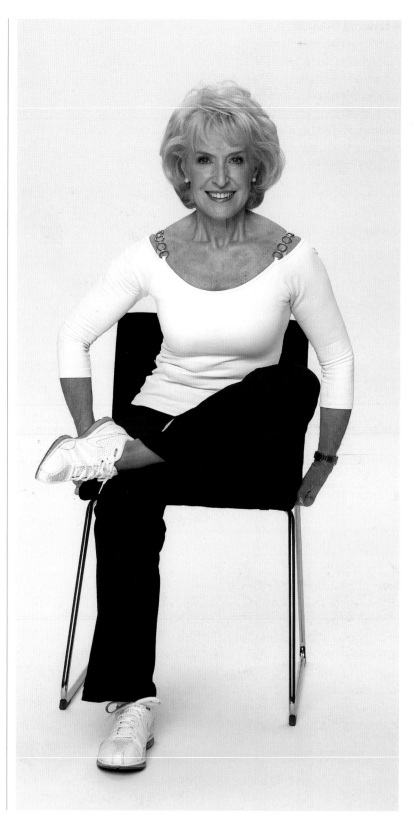

4 Front thigh stretch ▶

Stand and hold on to back of chair with right hand. Take left ankle in left hand (hold your trouser leg or sock if you find this difficult) and bring knees in line with each other, then press left hip forward to feel a stretch down front of thigh. Hold for 10 seconds, then change legs and repeat.

5 Bottom stretch ▶▶

Holding on to chair with right hand for support, bring left knee up and take hold under your left thigh. Stand up straight and bring knee closer to chest to feel a stretch in your bottom. Hold for 10 seconds, then change legs and repeat.

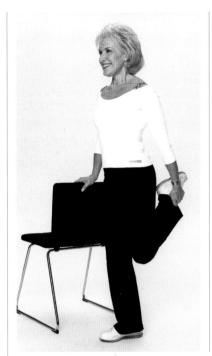
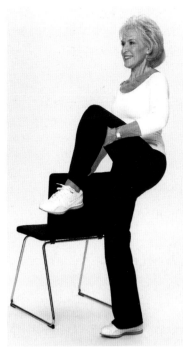

AEROBIC CHALLENGE

Walk up and down stairs 3 times consecutively. Do this 4 times in total throughout the day.

Exercise tip

Every bit of physical activity you do burns extra calories, so make an effort to move about more in your everyday life. Use the stairs more, park your car further away from the office or shops, take a walk at lunchtime, offer to carry bags and boxes for colleagues – it all adds up and will help you to lose weight faster.

MOTIVATIONAL THOUGHT FOR THE DAY

It can be really motivating to read how other people have succeeded in losing weight and turning their lives around. You'll find real-life slimming success stories in my *Diet & Fitness* magazine or you can watch the slimmers being interviewed on www.rosemaryconley.tv. One day these people resolved to do something about their weight, just like you. They decided enough was enough and that they were going to make some changes – and they did.

One of the most important factors that determines who is featured in the magazine is the quality of a slimmer's 'before' photograph. I know we hate having our photograph taken if we are overweight – I didn't even have one of myself when I was at my biggest – but it will demonstrate how far you have come once you have reached your goal weight. It is that dramatic transformation that inspires other potential dieters to take action. So, if you have not taken your before photograph yet, please do so today, before too many excess pounds and inches disappear!

Have you found yourself a notebook or folder for recording your notes and observations of how you feel? It's really good therapy as you progress on your weight loss journey as it will act as a constant reminder of your achievements.

Day 3

Every day is important but today is really important. It's the day your body starts drawing on its 'savings account' of fat to make up the deficit left by the reduction in your daily calories and the increase in your physical activity.

During the first couple of days of a diet, it's likely that your body is still processing some of the food you ate before you started the diet, alongside the restricted calories from this 14-Day Fast Track diet, and you will also be burning some of the carbohydrate stored in your liver and muscles. But from today, your body will only be using the calories from the food you are now eating to fuel essential bodily functions, and the resulting shortfall in calories needed for the extra activity you are doing is being drawn from your fat stores. So, from now on, you will be getting slimmer.

Eating your between-meals power snacks will help you get through the morning and afternoon without hunger pangs, but if you find you are not hungry at any of these times, save these calories for when you do feel like a nibble. For instance, I have my breakfast at 6.30 a.m. and I am always really hungry by lunchtime at 12.30 p.m., but then I can easily go right through to my next main meal at 7 p.m. without feeling hungry. However, I like to have a little something, usually a tiny portion of cereal, before I go to bed at 10 p.m. We are all different, so make the diet work for you.

Choose carefully from today's menu and enjoy your food. The toning exercises today will work on the abdominals, back, inner thighs, underarms and chest, and the aerobic activity will burn fat.

MENU

Breakfast
■ 1 Müllerlight yogurt, any flavour (max. 150 kcal), plus 1 small banana

Mid-morning power snack
■ 1 × 200g slice melon (weighed without skin) ✓

Lunch
■ 1 pitta bread, split open, then spread with low-fat Marie Rose dressing or very low-fat mayonnaise and filled with shredded lettuce, cherry tomatoes and 100g cooked prawns
OR
■ 1 × 300 pack Rosemary Conley Solo Slim Tomato Soup (order from www.rosemaryconley.com), plus 1 slice wholegrain bread ✓

Mid-afternoon power snack
■ 1 Rakusen's cracker topped with 1 × 20g triangle Laughing Cow Extra Light soft cheese, plus 5 cherry tomatoes

Dinner
■ Quick and Easy Chicken Curry: Dry-fry 1 × 115g chopped chicken breast (no skin) or Quorn chicken-style fillets in a preheated non-stick pan with ½ chopped onion and 1 crushed garlic clove. Sprinkle 1 tsp curry powder over and 'cook out' for 1 minute, then add 1 small chopped chilli, ½ chopped green pepper, 25g button mushrooms (optional) and 1 × 400g can chopped tomatoes, and simmer for 5 minutes to reduce. Serve with 1 blue Portion Pot® (55g uncooked weight) or 1 red Portion Pot® (144g cooked weight) basmati rice ✓
OR
■ Leek and Sage Meatballs with Pasta (see recipe, p.218) ✓

WARM-UP

Stair step-ups

Using a single step (such as the bottom step of your stairs or your front doorstep), step up and down for 2 minutes. Lead with the right leg for 1 minute, then pause and change to lead with the left leg. Make sure the whole foot makes contact on each step.

FIVE-MINUTE TONE-UP

1 Chest shaper ▶

(2 × 10 reps)

Lie on back with knees bent, holding a weight or water bottle in each hand, arms bent at right angles at sides and elbows in line with shoulders Ⓐ. Now breathe in and, as you breathe out, extend arms above chest without locking elbows Ⓑ. Lower again under control. Do 10 reps in total, then rest before doing another set.

2 Underarm toner ▶

(2 × 10 reps each arm)

Still lying on your back with knees bent, hold a weight or bottle in left hand and place hand by side of your head with elbow pointing towards ceiling. Support left arm with your other hand Ⓐ. Breathe in and, as you breathe out, extend left arm without locking elbow Ⓑ, then bend again, taking care to keep your head still. Do 10 reps, then change arms and repeat. Rest before doing another set.

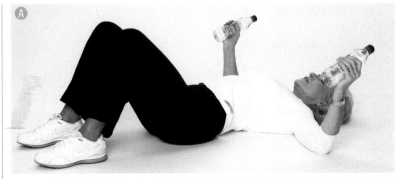

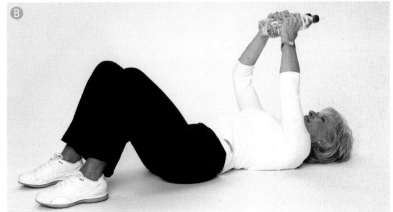

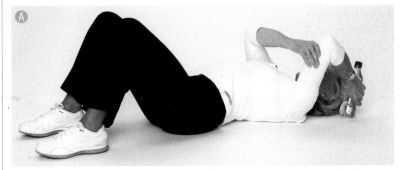

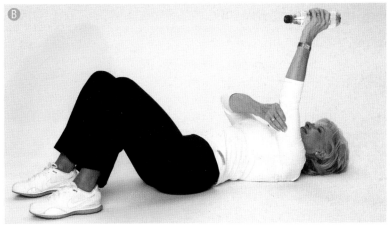

3 Inner thigh toner ▶

(2 × 8 reps)

Lying on back with knees bent, place a small, thick cushion between knees. Make sure feet are parallel and firmly planted on the floor. Now breathe in and, as you breathe out, squeeze cushion and hold for 3 seconds. Breathe in again as you release. Do 8 reps, then rest before doing another set.

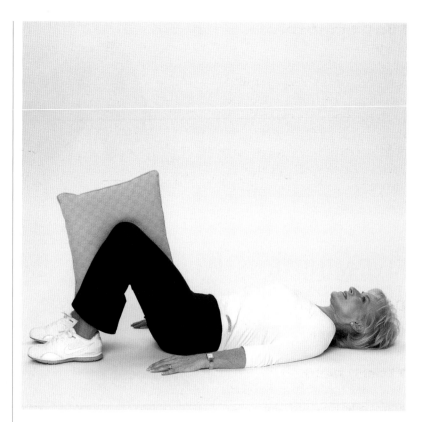

4 Tummy curl ▶

(2 × 10 reps)

Lying on back with knees bent and feet hip width apart, place right hand behind head and left hand on top of left thigh. Breathe in and, as you breathe out, lift head and shoulders off floor, pulling tummy in tight. Lower again slowly, keeping tummy in. Do 10 reps, then rest before doing another set.

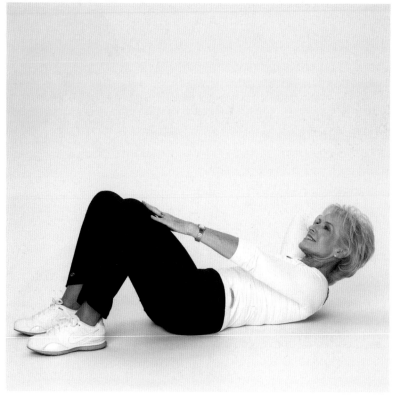

5 Back strengthener ▶

(2 × 6 reps)

Lie on front with both arms bent at right angles and elbows in line with shoulders Ⓐ. Breathe in and, as you breathe out, lift head and shoulders just off floor but keep head facing the floor Ⓑ. Pause for 2 seconds, then release. Do 6 reps, then rest before doing another set.

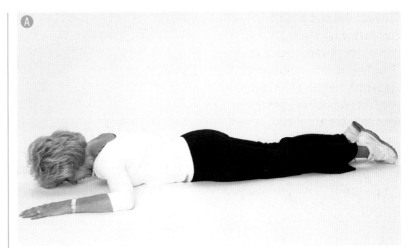

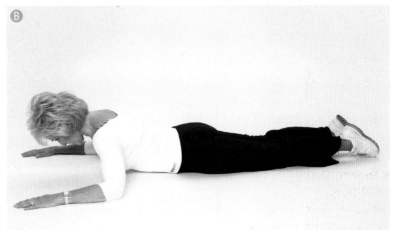

POST-WORKOUT STRETCHES

1 Tummy stretch ▼

Lie on front with arms at sides and elbows bent. Now prop up on your elbows, keeping your hips in contact with floor, and lift your chin forward slightly to feel a stretch in your tummy. Hold for 10 seconds, then release.

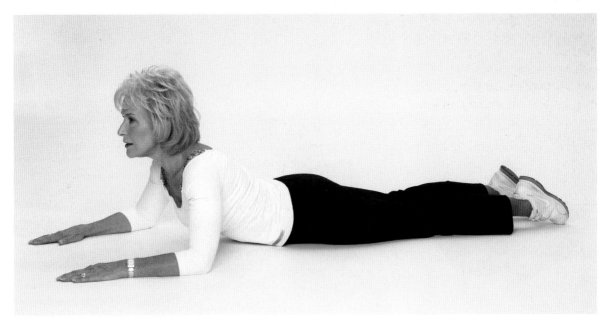

2 Back stretch ▶

Come up onto your hands and knees and, as you pull your tummy in, arch your spine up towards the ceiling, letting your head drop down. Hold for 10 seconds, then release.

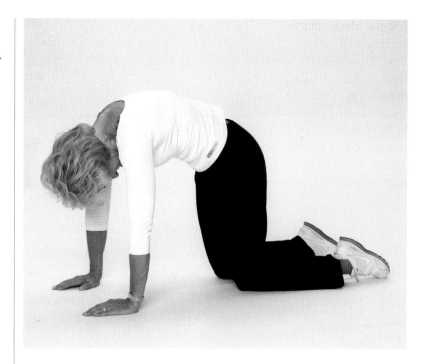

3 Underarm stretch ▼

Sit upright with legs crossed and place right hand behind right shoulder. Press left hand on your right underarm to push right hand further down your back. Keep your head up and look straight ahead. Hold for 10 seconds, then change arms and repeat.

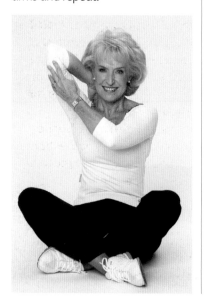

4 Chest stretch ▼

Sit upright and place hands behind you on the floor. Draw your shoulders back to feel a stretch across your chest. Hold for 10 seconds, then release.

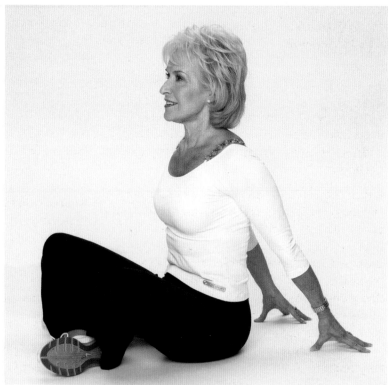

5 Inner thigh stretch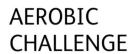

Sit upright with soles of feet together and elbows resting on inside of thighs. Keeping your head up and back straight, lean forward and press elbows onto thighs. Hold for 10 seconds, then breathe in and, as you breathe out, press down further on thighs and hold for another 10 seconds.

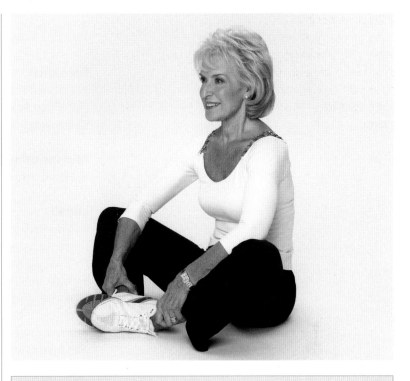

AEROBIC CHALLENGE

Work out at an aerobics class or to a fitness DVD for 30 minutes or go for a 30-minute walk.

Exercise tip

When doing strength exercises, always work your muscles to the point where they feel tired, then do five more reps. This way, you challenge the muscle fibres and they become stronger. It is these extra reps that do the real work.

MOTIVATIONAL THOUGHT FOR THE DAY

Writing down our goals and ambitions is really important if we are serious about achieving them, and it's the same when trying to lose weight and get fitter.

Back in the 1950s, the Board of Governors at Yale University in the US decided to survey all their final-year students to establish their lifestyles, eating habits, religious beliefs, hobbies, and so on. One of the questions asked was 'Do you have any goals?'. As this was one of the top universities in the US, the Board was somewhat surprised to learn that only 10 per cent of students admitted to having goals. Next, the questionnaire asked if the students had written down those goals. Only four per cent said they had.

Twenty years later, the university thought it would be interesting to find out how the original group of students had progressed since they completed the study 20 years earlier. It took a year to track them all down and one or two had died, but all those still living completed the new survey. The most interesting factor to emerge was that the four per cent who had said they had goals and had written them down, were *each* earning more than the *total* earnings of the remaining 96 per cent!

So, determine your goals and write them down. It works! You can always revise your goals, add to them, and remove any that become unimportant, but having a goal to aim for keeps you focused and helps to keep you on track.

Day 4

You should be feeling slimmer today. When you woke up this morning did your stomach feel a little flatter? And when you got dressed, hopefully your waistband felt less tight and your clothes looser. It's a great feeling!

The temptation at this point is to think that you have the diet sussed and that you don't need to measure the quantities of food you eat, but trust me, you do. Portion control will make a big difference to your overall rate of weight and inch loss. If you don't already own a set of my Portion Pots®, check them out on www.rosemaryconley.com. They are unique, inexpensive and incredibly effective. And if you join one of our classes or our online club, you will receive a set free in your membership pack.

Today's toning exercises focus on the waist, stomach, backside and outer thighs and your posture muscles in the upper back. Be as active as you can and stick strictly to the diet plan. If you do, the rewards will be fantastic.

MENU

Breakfast
■ 1 yellow Portion Pot® (125ml) fresh orange juice, plus 1 slice wholegrain bread spread with 2 tsps marmalade, jam or honey ☑

Mid-morning power snack
■ 2 dried apricots ☑

Lunch
■ 2 low-fat beef or pork sausages (max. 5% fat) or 2 Quorn sausages, grilled, served with 1 yellow Portion Pot® (115g) baked beans, 1 dry-fried small egg, 1 small can tomatoes boiled well to reduce, plus unlimited grilled or boiled mushrooms ☑ P
OR
■ Chicken Noodle Soup (see recipe, p.211) served with 1 small wholegrain pitta bread, toasted

Mid-afternoon power snack
■ 1 kiwi fruit plus 5 seedless grapes ☑

Dinner
■ Chinese Chicken Kebabs (see recipe, p.211) served with 1 blue Portion Pot® (55g uncooked weight) or 1 red Portion Pot® (144g cooked weight) basmati rice per person
OR
■ 1 low-fat pizza (max. 350 kcal and 5% fat, e.g. Marks & Spencer Count On Us) served with a mixed salad tossed in fat-free dressing ☑

WARM-UP

March on spot with tummy pull-ins
Stand tall and march on the spot, letting the arms swing naturally. Every 10 steps, really pull your tummy in tight and then relax it for 10 steps. This is a great tummy flattener that you can do throughout the day!

FIVE-MINUTE TONE-UP

1 Waist twist ▶

(2 × 8 reps alternate sides)
Lie on back with knees bent, feet
flat on floor, and place both hands
behind head. Breathe in and, as
you breathe out, pull your tummy
in and lift head and shoulders off
floor, bringing right hand across
body towards opposite knee. Keep
your chin off your chest as you lift.
Lower again, bringing hand back
behind head, then lift to other side.
Change sides for 8 reps, then rest
before doing another set.

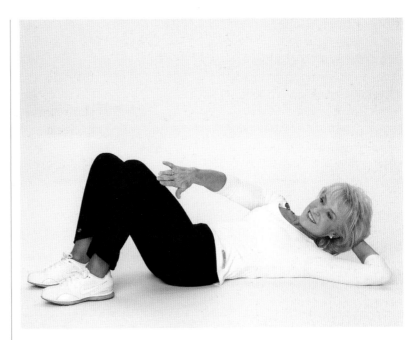

2 Reverse tummy curl ▶

(2 × 6 reps)
Still lying on your back, bring knees
towards chest and cross your
ankles. Place palms of hands face
down on floor and pull tummy in
tight Ⓐ. Breathe in and, as you
breathe out, lift hips off floor,
bringing knees closer to your chest
Ⓑ. Keep your neck and shoulders
relaxed and gently push hands
against the floor for support. Do 6
reps slowly, then rest with feet on
the floor before doing another set.

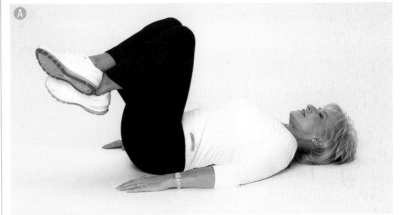

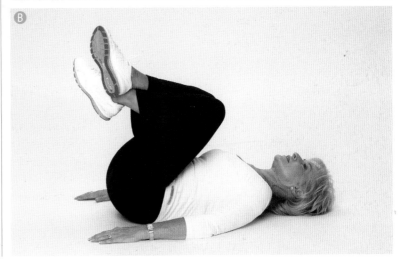

3 Outer thigh shaper ▶

(2 × 12 reps each leg)

Lie on side, bend your bottom leg
up to 90 degrees and push top leg
out straight in line with hip, foot
flexed. Hold a weight or water
bottle on the thigh Ⓐ. Pull tummy
in to hold trunk still, then lift top leg
under control Ⓑ and lower again.
Do 12 reps, then roll over and
repeat with other leg. Rest before
doing another set.

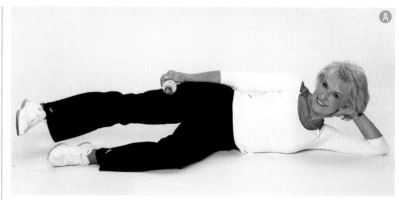

4 Bottom shaper ▼

(2 × 8 reps alternate legs)

Lie on front with legs wider than
hip width and feet turned out
slightly. Pull your tummy in, then
lift and lower alternate legs under
control. Keep your upper body very
relaxed at all times. Do 8 reps (4
each side), then rest before doing
another set.

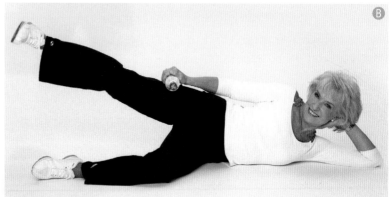

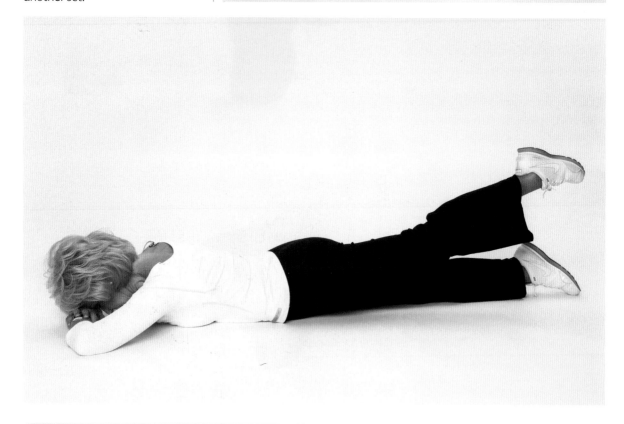

5 Posture improver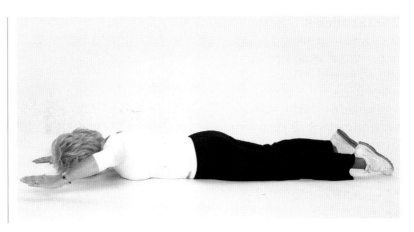

(2 × 6 reps alternate arms)
Still lying on front, place both arms out to sides at right angles with elbows in line with shoulders and shoulders down. Keeping your head down and relaxed, lift bent left arm off floor (if this is too difficult, just lift elbow). Lower again, then lift other arm. Keep changing sides for 6 reps, then rest before repeating another set.

POST-WORKOUT STRETCHES

1 Upper back stretch ▶

Sit up tall with legs crossed, then bring both arms forward at shoulder height and clasp hands. Drop your head forward to feel a stretch in back of neck, then gently press upper back away from your hands to feel a stretch in upper back. Hold for 10 seconds, then release.

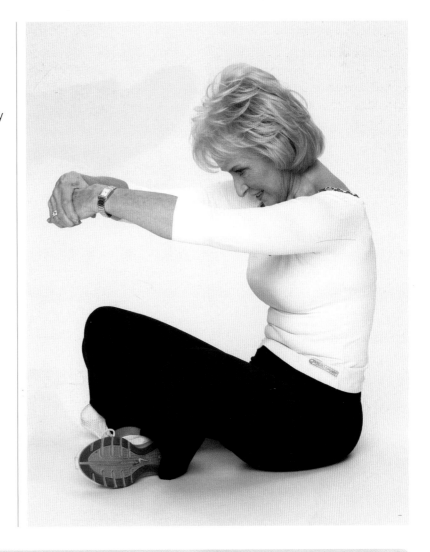

2 Waist stretch ▶

Sit up tall, lift your right arm and lean over to left side, keeping both hips on the floor and without leaning forward or back. Hold for 10 seconds, then change sides.

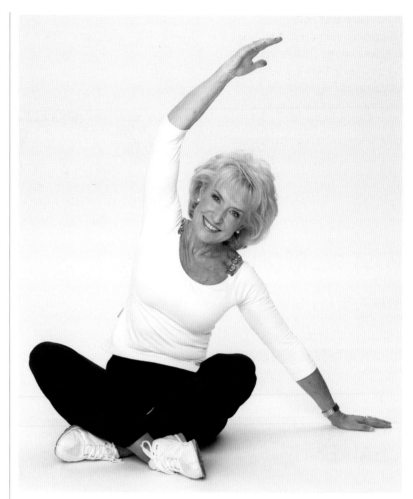

3 Outer thigh and hip ▶ stretch

Sit upright with legs straight out in front and bring left foot over right leg, placing foot flat on floor. Place left hand on floor for support and right hand across left knee. Use pressure of right arm to pull left leg further across body to feel a stretch in outer thigh and hip. Hold for 10 seconds, then change legs and repeat.

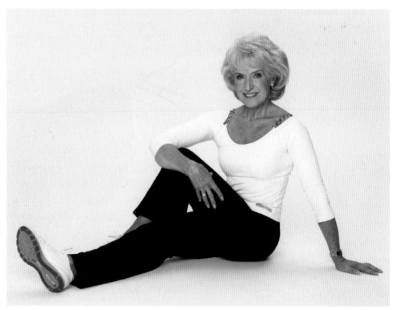

4 Bottom stretch ▶

Lie on back with knees bent and feet flat on floor. Take hold behind both knees and bring them closer to your chest to stretch the back of your hips. Keep head on floor and keep neck and shoulders relaxed. Hold for 10 seconds, then release.

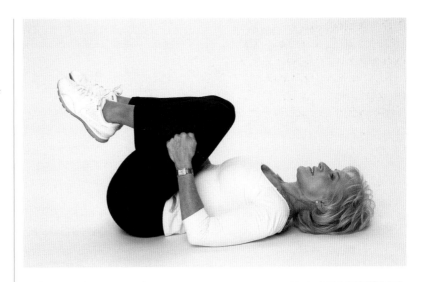

5 Tummy stretch ▶

Straighten your legs and take arms overhead. Stretch arms away from legs to feel a stretch down your tummy. Hold for 10 seconds, then release.

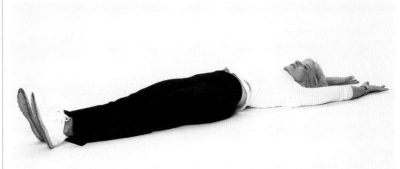

AEROBIC CHALLENGE

Go for a cycle ride for 20 minutes or cycle on a stationary exercise bike for 10 minutes, plus either walk briskly for 10 minutes at some point in the day or go for a 20-minute swim.

Exercise tip

If you watch television in the evening, why not use the time during the ad breaks or the breaks between programmes to walk up and down stairs three times. Do this four times in an evening and it will burn a significant number of calories and tone your bottom too!

MOTIVATIONAL THOUGHT FOR THE DAY

Research has shown that keeping a written record of what we eat and drink can affect how much weight we lose. In trials, slimmers who wrote down what they ate and drank, lost twice as much weight as those who didn't.

The reason why keeping a written record is so helpful is because it makes us accountable. We can very conveniently forget what we've eaten and swear blind that we have been saintly with our dieting regime, convincing ourselves that we really have! Writing down what you eat, as you eat it, is a great habit to get into and it will help you to understand your temptations and identify the times when you are most vulnerable to straying from the diet. It's for this reason that I have created a 'Handbook' to accompany this diet in which you write down everything you eat and drink, and the exercise you do, so you can then look back and see why you did so well one week and not on another. It's well worth the investment of effort.

Day 5

Well done for getting this far on the 14-Day Fast Track. If you are still sticking strictly to the diet and the exercises, you stand an extremely high chance of long-term success. If you were going to fail, you would have fallen by the wayside yesterday.

Three or four days into a diet is when slimmers are likely to feel peckish on occasions and not make time for the exercises. They may also be missing some of their favourite fattening foods or alcohol. However, if you want to regain your youthful figure and feel years younger in the next month or two, it's going to take determination, dedication and discipline. It's not difficult, though, if you have the right attitude and the will to succeed. The rewards for staying focused and disciplined are huge and I want you to picture yourself succeeding and looking fabulous in that new outfit you are going to wear when you reach your goal.

Today I'm giving you a rest from the toning exercises, but I would like you to do some extra aerobic exercise to boost your fat burning and weight loss. Look at my suggestions and select an activity you enjoy and don't forget to drink plenty of water before, during and after exercising.

Remember, nothing tastes as good as being slim feels!

MENU

Breakfast
- 1 slice wholegrain bread, toasted, topped with 1 yellow Portion Pot® (115g) baked beans ☑

Mid-morning power snack
- 1 blue Portion Pot® (14g) Special K cereal (eaten dry or with milk from allowance) ☑

Lunch
- Large salad of grated carrots, beansprouts, chopped peppers, celery, tomatoes, cucumber and red onion, served with 130g canned tuna chunks (in brine) or 1 blue Portion Pot® (100g) low-fat cottage cheese, plus 1 tbsp Hellmann's Extra Light Mayonnaise. Plus 1 low-fat yogurt (max. 100 kcal and 5% fat) ☑ P

Mid-afternoon power snack
- 100g cherries ☑

Dinner
- Chilli Prawn Stir-Fry with Peppers and Mushrooms: Dry-fry 150g fresh prawns in a non-stick wok. When they have changed colour, add ½ each chopped red and green pepper, 5 button mushrooms, 1 chopped celery stick, ½ chopped red onion, 1 small courgette, chopped, and ½ pack of fresh (or 1 whole can) beansprouts. Do not overcook. Just before serving add 1 tbsp Thai sweet chilli dipping sauce and soy sauce to taste P
Plus 1 low-fat yogurt or other low-fat dessert (max. 100 kcal and 5% fat)
OR
- Ham, Leek and Sweet Potato Pie (see recipe, p.216) with unlimited vegetables (excluding potatoes) or salad
OR
- Leek and Sage Meatballs with Pasta (see recipe, p.218) ☑

WARM-UP

Knee lifts with pull-downs

Stand upright with arms above head and tummy pulled in. Lift alternate knees and as you lift each knee, pull your arms down to either side of the knees. Keep your tummy in and your back straight and continue for 1 minute.

AEROBIC CHALLENGE

Exercise aerobically for a minimum of 30 minutes today. Select one of the following or create a combination of activities that you can do one after the other for 30 minutes in total:

- Swimming
- Brisk walking
- Cycling
- Aerobics (class or DVD)
- Heavy housework (vacuuming, cleaning windows, bed making, etc.)
- Cardio equipment in the gym (e.g. stepper, cross trainer, bike, treadmill)

Warm up first and then, after your chosen activity, cool down by just gently walking on the spot for 2 minutes, then stretch out at the end of your workout to avoid aching muscles tomorrow.

POST-AEROBIC STRETCHES

Do these stretches in the order shown as they work together very well. Hold each stretch for about 10 seconds.

1 Calf stretch ▼

Place one foot in front of the other, with both feet pointing forward (hold on to a wall or sturdy surface for support if you wish). Bend front knee in line with ankle and keep back leg straight with heel pressing down flat on the floor. Lean further forward to feel a stretch in calf of back leg and hold for 10 seconds. Do the lower calf stretch (exercise 2, p.48) before changing legs.

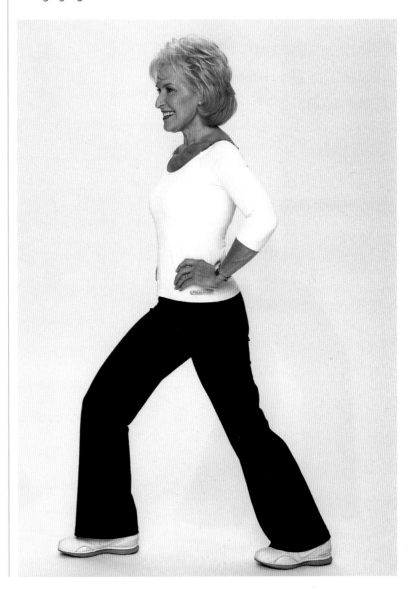

2 Lower calf stretch ▼

Bring your back foot half a step in and bend both knees with feet still pointing forward. Keep both heels on floor and your body upright as you look straight ahead and hold for 10 seconds. Change legs and repeat both calf stretches.

3 Back thigh stretch ▼

Straighten your front leg and keep your back leg bent. With spine straight, lean forward slightly to feel a stretch in back thigh of straight leg. Hold for 10 seconds, then change legs and repeat.

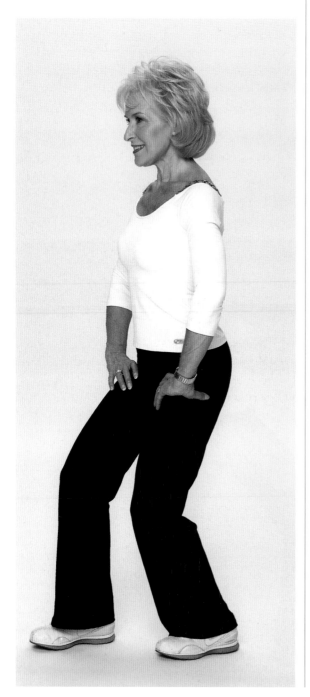

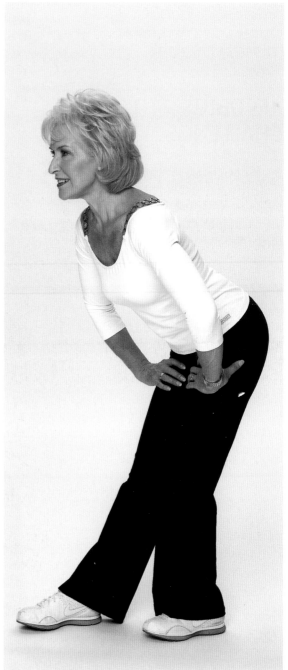

4 Front of hip stretch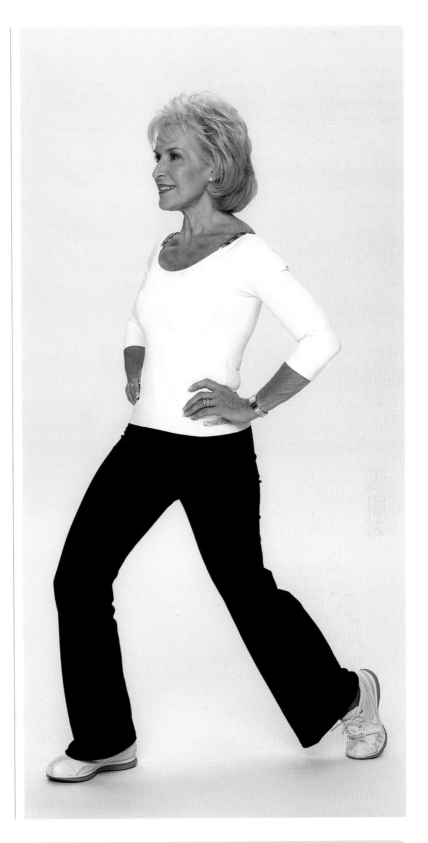

Bend front leg and lift heel of back foot. With your weight equally distributed between both legs, trunk upright and tummy in, press pelvis forward to feel a stretch at top of hip. Hold for 10 seconds, then change legs and repeat.

5 Front thigh stretch ▶

Stand upright and take hold of one ankle with hand (place other hand on wall or back of chair for support if necessary). Bring knees in line with each other and keep supporting leg slightly bent. Gently push hip of raised leg forward to stretch front of thigh. Hold stretch for 10 seconds, then change legs and repeat.

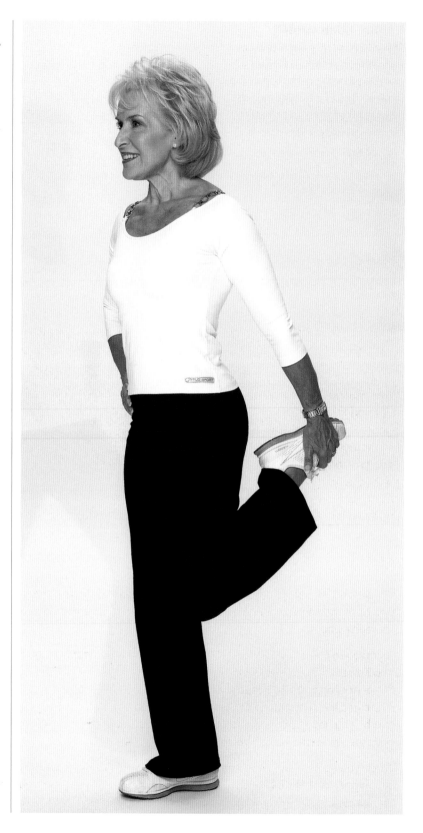

6 Inner thigh stretch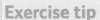

Stand tall and take legs out wide. Bend one knee in line with ankle, keeping other leg straight with foot pointing forward, to feel a stretch in inner thigh of straight leg. Hold for 10 seconds, then change legs and repeat.

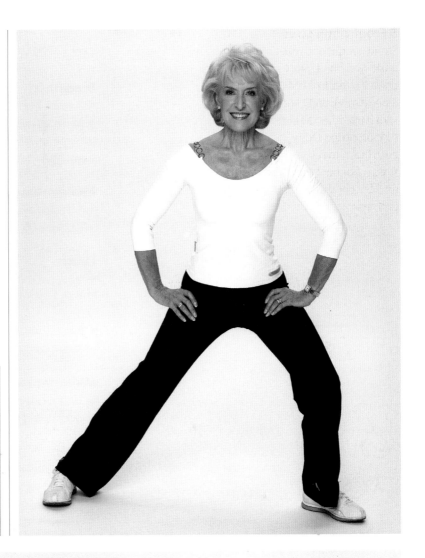

Exercise tip

When you go for a walk, include a few jogging steps every hundred yards, then walk again for another hundred yards. Turn your walk into a walk/jog and you will burn significantly more calories and see a dramatic improvement in your fitness.

MOTIVATIONAL THOUGHT FOR THE DAY

We all need encouragement when aiming for a goal and never more so than when we are trying to lose weight. It may be that your husband or partner is a real 'encourager', but if they aren't, you need to find someone who is!

If you go to one of our diet and fitness classes you will be surrounded by encouragers and that could be a good place to find a diet buddy. For members of our online club, the online chatroom and coffee shop offer the perfect opportunity for encouraging each other. Alternatively, you might find someone at work who is interested in your progress and will help to support and encourage you when the going gets tough, or maybe you have a mum or sister who will be brilliant at the job. It doesn't matter who it is, as long as you have someone who is positive and interested in you.

When you do find your encourager, explain to them how much you value their interest and encouragement. We all like to feel needed but we don't like to overstep the mark, so it's important to let the encourager know how much they are appreciated and that they are doing a useful job.

Day 6

After today, there's only one more day to go before the first week's weigh-in. Now is the time to be extra vigilant at avoiding temptation and to work especially hard at the exercises. I have increased the intensity of the exercises today so that you burn extra calories and fat. This is now the big push to maximum weight and inch loss at the beginning of Day 8.

Don't be tempted to skip meals as you will only end up feeling so hungry you'll be tempted to grab anything to eat! So eat your meals and your Power Snacks and do your exercises. Today's five-minute tone-up will work on your waist, back, inner and front thighs and your chest. If you stick to the diet and do the exercises, I PROMISE you will lose weight. Have a good day.

MENU

Breakfast
- 1 yellow Portion Pot® (30g) fruit and fibre cereal served with milk from allowance and topped with 1 red Portion Pot® (115g) fresh raspberries or 1 tsp sugar ☑

Mid-morning power snack
- 1 Ryvita spread thinly with Philadelphia Extra Light soft cheese ☑

Lunch
- 1 pre-packed sandwich of your choice (max. 300 kcal and 5 % fat) ☑
OR
- Broccoli and Leek Soup (see recipe, p.210) served with a small granary roll ☑

Mid-afternoon power snack
- 10 cherry tomatoes, plus chunks of carrots, cucumber and pepper ☑

Dinner
- Spicy Chicken Pasta: Dry-fry 110g chopped chicken breast (no skin) and ½ chopped onion in a non-stick wok and season with freshly ground black pepper. Add 1 crushed garlic clove, 1 sliced green pepper, 1 × 400g can chopped tomatoes, ½ small chopped chilli and a dash of Worcestershire sauce and allow to simmer for 5 minutes. Serve with 1 yellow Portion Pot® (45g uncooked weight) or 1 red Portion Pot® (110g cooked weight) pasta shapes
OR
- Sweet and Sour Quorn: Dry-fry ½ × 350g pack Quorn Chicken Style Pieces (175g) with ½ chopped onion, ½ each chopped red and green pepper, 5 button mushrooms, halved, 1 chopped celery stick and 1 small chopped courgette ☑ℙ
Plus 1 low-fat yogurt or other dessert (max. 100 kcal and 5 % fat)

WARM-UP

Pretend skipping

Imagine you are holding a skipping rope. Begin a small bounce on the spot as you pretend to turn the rope. You can turn around in a circle and even do some fancy arm work such as figure 8s!

FIVE-MINUTE TONE-UP

1 Waist toner

(2 × 12 reps alternate sides)
Stand upright with feet parallel and hip width apart and knees slightly bent. Hold a weight or water bottle in each hand and take both arms

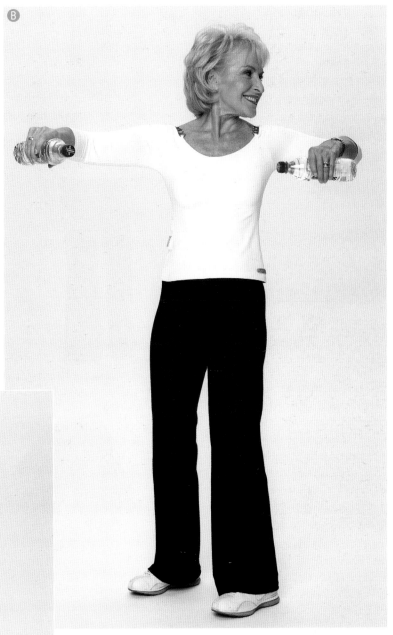

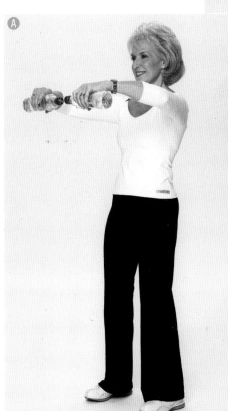

out in front at shoulder height Ⓐ. Now pull left elbow back, bending the arm and keeping it at shoulder height, with shoulders down and relaxed Ⓑ. Keep watching the elbow so your head turns as well, but make sure hips stay facing front. Bring arm forward again and repeat with other arm. Do 12 reps (6 each side), then rest before doing another set.

2 Thigh shaper ▶

(2 × 12 reps)

Keep feet parallel and bring arms down by sides, still holding weights or water bottles Ⓐ. Now, keeping knees hip width apart, bend knees and push hips back as if about to sit in a chair Ⓑ. Lift again and keep repeating for 12 reps, then rest before doing another set.

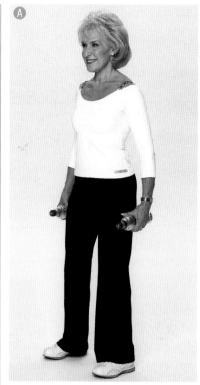
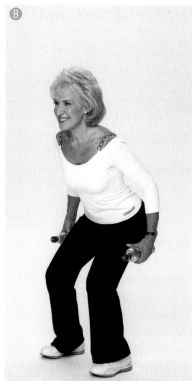

3 Chest shaper ▶

(2 × 12 reps)

Lie on back with knees bent, with a weight or water bottle in each hand, arms bent at right angles at your sides and elbows in line with shoulders Ⓐ. Now breathe in and, as you breathe out, extend arms above chest without locking elbows Ⓑ. Lower again under control and do 12 reps in total, then rest before doing another set.

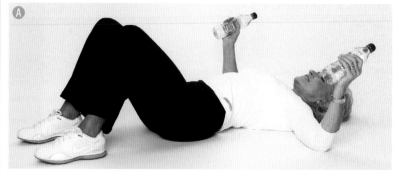
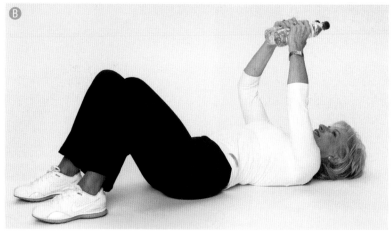

4 Inner thigh toner ▶

(2 × 10 reps)

Still lying on back with knees bent, place a small, thick cushion between knees. Make sure feet are parallel and firmly planted on the floor. Now breathe in and, as you breathe out, squeeze cushion to work inner thigh muscles and hold for 3 seconds. Breathe in again as you release. Do 10 reps, then rest before doing another set.

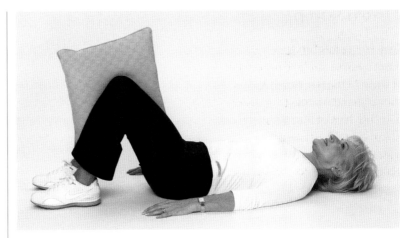

5 Back strengthener ▶▼

(2 × 8 reps)

Lie on front with both arms bent at right angles and elbows in line with shoulders Ⓐ. Breathe in and, as you breathe out, lift head and shoulders just off floor but keep your head facing the floor Ⓑ. Pause for 2 seconds then release. Do 8 reps, then rest before doing another set.

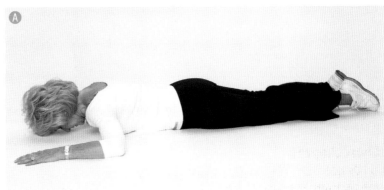

Ⓐ

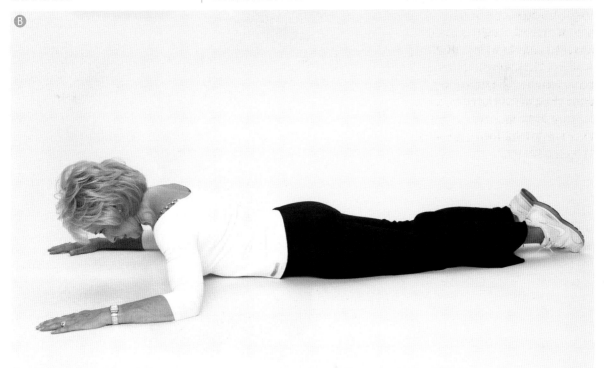

Ⓑ

POST-WORKOUT STRETCHES

1 Front thigh stretch ▶

Lie on your front, bend one knee and take hold of foot with hand on same side (if this is uncomfortable, just bend the knee). Keeping knees together, gently press hip into floor for 10 seconds, then release. Change legs and repeat.

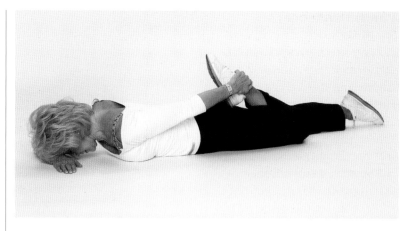

2 Spine stretch ▶

Come up onto hands and knees and, as you pull your tummy in, arch your spine up towards ceiling, letting your head drop down. Hold for 10 seconds, then release.

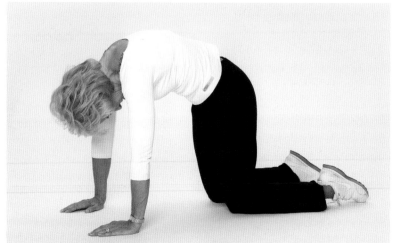

3 Chest stretch ▶

Sit upright and place both hands behind you on floor. Draw shoulders back to feel a stretch across chest, and hold for 10 seconds.

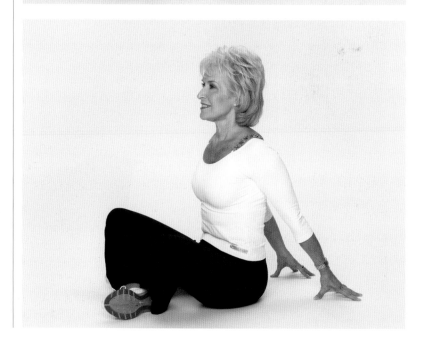

4 Waist stretch ▶

Sit up tall with legs crossed, then lift right arm and lean over to the left side, keeping both hips on floor and not leaning forward or back. Hold for 10 seconds, then change sides and repeat.

5 Inner thigh stretch ▼

Sit upright with soles of feet together and elbows resting on inside of thighs. Keeping your head up and back straight, lean forward and press elbows onto thighs. Hold for 10 seconds, then breathe in and, as you breathe out, press down further on thighs and hold for another 10 seconds.

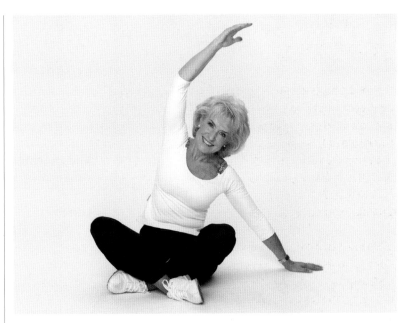

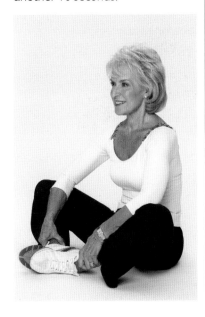

AEROBIC CHALLENGE

Take a brisk walk for 30 minutes at some point during the day.

Exercise tip

When doing toning or strength exercises, always breathe out on the 'effort', e.g. when lifting your head and shoulders on an abdominal curl, and breathe in as you return to the start position. And remember to keep breathing! Holding your breath for more than just a few seconds when exerting yourself can be dangerous.

MOTIVATIONAL THOUGHT FOR THE DAY

Be watchful of the temptation to sabotage your dieting efforts and find an excuse for breaking your diet and fitness programme. This is a common trait in people who are frightened of failing. If you have tried to lose weight before but didn't get the results you'd hoped for, you might be tempted to overeat or drink too much alcohol just before weighing day so you can say, 'Well I would have lost much more, but I had to go to Caroline's birthday celebration and that's why I've not lost as much as I should have.' Deliberately – though often subconsciously – ruining your chances of success is very destructive.

The diet will work if you stick to it and the exercises will tone you up and burn fat so that you lose fat and inches. Please trust the diet and don't even consider sabotaging your progress. Stay focused and think about how you will feel at the end of the programme if you stick to it, and the scales will reward you. The bonus is that you will gain confidence, which will help you as you progress towards your goal. You really have nothing to lose but your weight and inches, so go for it!

Day 7

Well done for reaching this stage. With your weighing and measuring day coming up tomorrow you need to put every bit of effort into the exercises in order to maximise your success on the scales first thing in the morning.

Today's diet offers lots of bulk as I don't want you feeling hungry and being tempted off track. Your body is now in full fat-burning mode, so every bit of willpower you can summon will pay dividends. Should you get hungry and be tempted to stray, remember that your body is drawing calories out of its savings account of fat.

Before my evening meal I always have two large glasses of diet ginger beer. I love it and it curbs my appetite so that I'm not overly hungry when I sit down to eat my main meal of the day. It works for me. If you are really hungry by the time you start eating, you'll find the amount of time it takes you to eat your meal isn't long enough for the food to reach your stomach and register that you've had enough. So try to eat slowly and drink plenty of water or low-calorie drinks to allow time for your brain to receive that 'I'm full' signal.

Today's toning exercises are more challenging and are designed to work the muscles in your waist, abdomen, backside, outer thighs and underarms. Your muscles are becoming stronger every day, so feel the muscles 'working' as you do each exercise.

MENU

Breakfast
- 2 Quorn sausages, grilled, served with 1 medium-sized dry-fried egg and 1 × 200g can tomatoes, boiled until reduced ✓ P

Mid-morning power snack
- 20g sultanas ✓

Lunch
- 200g 2% fat Greek yogurt mixed with 1 tsp runny honey and 1 red Portion Pot® (115g) raspberries or chopped strawberries or 1 yellow Portion Pot® (70g) blueberries, topped with 1 tsp muesli ✓
OR
- Greek Salad Wrap (see recipe, p.222) ✓

Mid-afternoon power snack
- 100g fresh pineapple ✓

Dinner
- 150g roast chicken breast (no skin) served with 100g dry-roast sweet potatoes plus 200g other vegetables of your choice (e.g. carrots, broccoli, cauliflower) and low-fat gravy
OR
- 2 Quorn Lamb Style Grills, grilled, served with 115g boiled new potatoes (with skins), plus 200g other vegetables of your choice and a little low-fat gravy and mint sauce ✓

WARM-UP

Twisted canoeing

Stand tall and take both arms above head with tummy in. Now lower both arms to one side as you bend knees and hips, then come up again and repeat, dropping arms to other side. Imagine you are canoeing down a river! Keep going for 1 minute.

FIVE-MINUTE TONE-UP

1 Tummy curl ▶

(2 × 10 reps)

Lie on back with both hands behind head, knees bent and feet hip width apart Ⓐ. Now breathe in and, as you breathe out, lift head and shoulders off floor, pulling your navel in towards your spine Ⓑ. Keep your chin off your chest and look forward as you lift. Do 10 reps, then rest before doing another set.

2 Waist twist ▶

(2 × 12 reps alternate sides)

Still lying on back with knees bent, place both hands behind head. Breathe in and, as you breathe out, pull tummy in and lift head and shoulders off floor, bringing right hand across towards left knee and keeping chin off chest. Lower again, bringing hand back behind head, then lift to other side. Change sides for 12 reps (6 each side), then rest before doing another set.

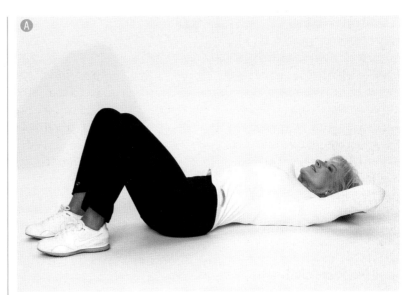

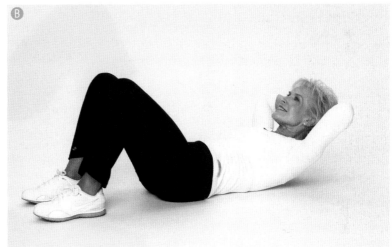

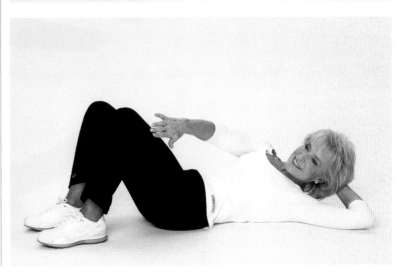

3 Underarm toner ▶

(2 × 12 reps each arm)
Lying as before, hold a weight or bottle in left hand and place hand by side of your head with elbow pointing towards ceiling. Support left arm with your other hand Ⓐ. Breathe in and, as you breathe out, extend left arm without locking elbow Ⓑ then bend it again, taking care to keep your head still. Do 12 reps, then change arms and repeat. Rest before doing another set.

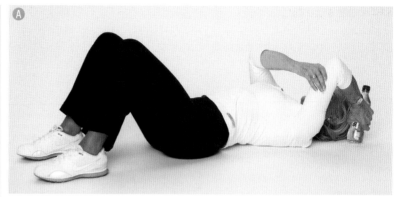

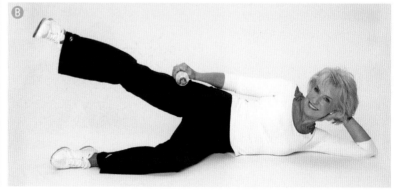

4 Outer thigh shaper ▶

(× 16 reps each leg)
Lie on side, bend bottom leg up to 90 degrees and push top leg out straight in line with hip, with foot flexed. Hold a weight or water bottle on the thigh Ⓐ. Pull tummy in to hold trunk still, then lift top leg under control Ⓑ and slowly lower again. Keep lifting and lowering leg for 16 reps, then roll over and repeat with other leg.

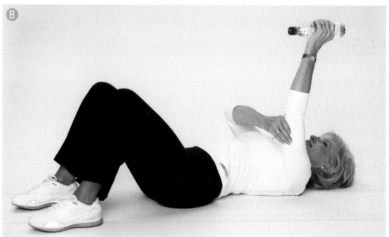

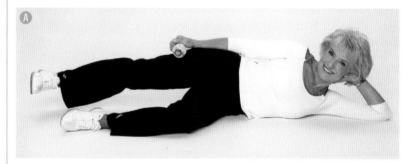

5 Bottom shaper ▶

(2 × 4 reps each leg)
Lie on front with legs wider than hip width and feet turned out slightly. Pull tummy in and lift and lower one leg under control 4 times, then change legs and repeat. Rest before doing another set. Keep your upper body very relaxed at all times.

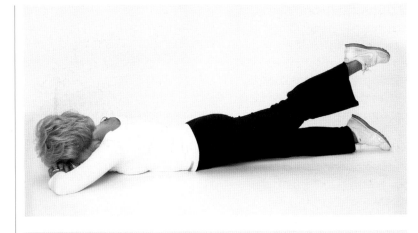

POST-WORKOUT STRETCHES

1 Waist stretch ▶

Sit up tall with legs crossed. Lift right arm and lean over to the left side, keeping both hips on the floor and without leaning forward or back. Hold for 10 seconds, then change sides and repeat.

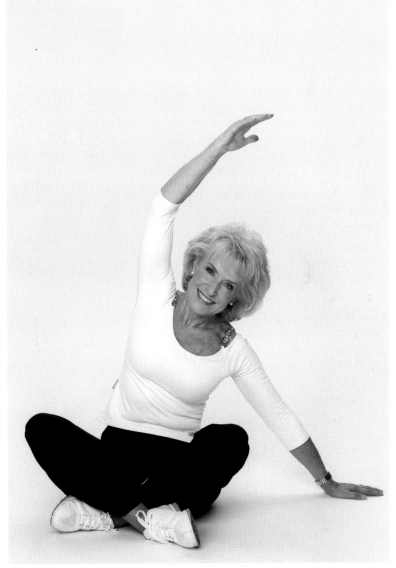

2 Outer thigh and hip ▶ stretch

Sit upright with legs straight out in front and bring left foot over right leg, placing foot flat on floor. Place left hand on floor for support and right hand across left knee. Use pressure of right arm to pull left leg further across body to feel a stretch in outer thigh and hip. Hold for 10 seconds, then change legs and repeat.

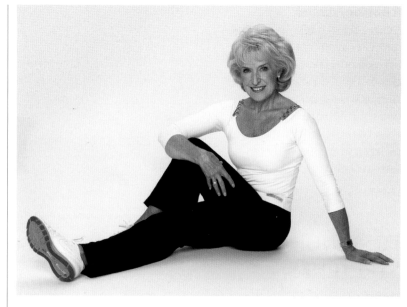

3 Underarm stretch ▶

Sit upright with legs crossed and place right hand behind right shoulder. Press left hand on right underarm to push right hand further down your back. Keep your head up and look straight ahead. Hold for 10 seconds, then change arms and repeat.

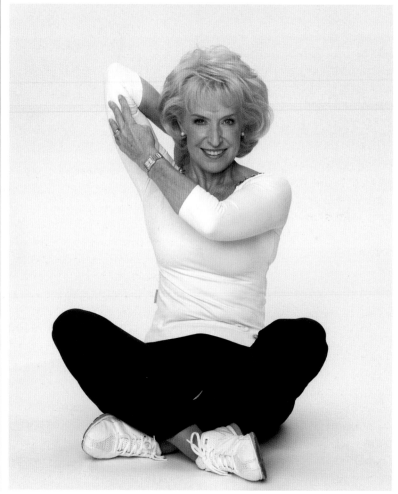

4 Bottom stretch ▶

Lie on back with both knees bent and feet flat on floor. Take hold behind both knees and bring them closer to your chest to stretch the back of your hips. Keep your neck and shoulders relaxed and your head on the floor. Hold for 10 seconds, then release.

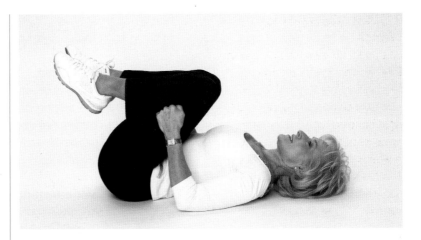

5 Tummy stretch ▶

Lie on back, straighten legs and take arms overhead. Stretch arms away from legs to feel a stretch down your tummy. Hold for 10 seconds, then release.

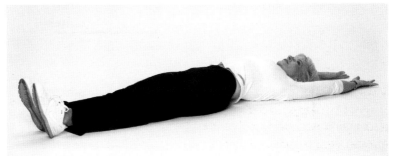

AEROBIC CHALLENGE

Go for a brisk 30-minute walk or work out to a fitness DVD for 30 minutes. Also, walk up and down stairs 4 times consecutively, twice during the day. Really go for it today!

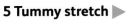

Exercise tip

It's important to have some water close by when exercising. Taking regular top-ups of water during aerobic exercise has been proven to be very effective in helping us to keep going for longer, for instance when exercising on a treadmill or exercise bike.

MOTIVATIONAL THOUGHT FOR THE DAY

Having reached this stage, you have taken a very big step towards a new you. Starting a diet and fitness campaign properly prepared, and then completing the first week, is a major achievement. The delight you will feel tomorrow when you step on the scales will give you an enormous boost and this will set you up for the next seven days. After you have completed the 14-Day Fast Track your calorie allowance will be increased according to your age, gender and weight, but sticking to the 1200-calorie allowance during this first phase of the diet will give you a fantastic start in your weight loss campaign. Research has shown that if we make significant progress early in our dieting campaign, we are far more likely to continue on the diet because we have already witnessed the inches disappearing and our clothes are feeling looser.

Make a real effort with the exercises today. I have given you some additional aerobic fat-burning activities to help you burn extra calories and fat and maximise the results for tomorrow. If you want to do even more, that's great. Stick to the diet, watch your portion sizes and don't cheat! You'll be so glad tomorrow.

Day 8

By the time you read this you will already have weighed and measured yourself. Make sure you write down your results. Try on your measuring belt and mark on it your new waist measurement. If you have a Magic Measure®, clip on your second set of tags and see how much you are shrinking. Add up the total number of inches (or centimetres) you have lost and look at the equivalent measurement on a ruler. It is fascinating to see the inches end to end in a straight line!

Hopefully, you will have lost a significant amount of weight too. Now find yourself a carrier bag and place in it some tins of food or packets of dried food of the equivalent weight that you have lost this week. Keep them in that bag and stash it away in a cupboard or under the stairs to be brought out this time next week or any time in between when you need a motivational boost and a reminder of what you have achieved so far.

Just one more week to go on this very strict diet. Stick with it and you will be the winner! Today's toning exercises will work your abdominals a little harder than before. I have also included an exercise that works your backside and your inner thighs at the same time and another that works your chest and underarms simultaneously, plus one for your shoulders and one for your back. Don't rush them but do them carefully to make them more effective. I've given you a break from your aerobic exercise today, so enjoy the rest!

Remember, all meals in each category are interchangeable.

MENU

Breakfast
■ Tomatoes and Mushrooms on Toast: Boil 1 × 400g can chopped tomatoes well to reduce to a thick consistency and season well with freshly ground black pepper. Spoon onto 1 large slice toasted wholegrain bread and serve with 10 grilled mushrooms ☑

Mid-morning power snack
■ 1 red Portion Pot® (115g) raspberries topped with 2 tsps low-fat yogurt ☑

Lunch
■ 2 hard-boiled eggs served with salad of chopped vegetables and salad leaves, tossed in low-fat dressing of your choice. Plus 1 kiwi fruit and 1 small pear ☑ 🅿
OR
■ Turkey and Mango Samosas (see recipe, p.213) served with unlimited fresh vegetables or salad

Mid-afternoon power snack
■ 150g fresh fruit salad ☑

Dinner
■ Beef Kebabs: Cut 150g rump steak into bite-sized pieces and thread on to wooden skewers with 8 chestnut mushrooms, then baste with 50g tomato passata and 1 tsp balti curry paste. Cook the kebabs for 5–6 minutes in a health grill or 10 minutes under a conventional grill. Check the centre of meat is cooked and, when ready to serve, sprinkle with ½ tbsp chopped fresh coriander and serve with fresh green vegetables or salad 🅿
OR
■ Any low-fat ready meal (max. 400 kcal and 5 % fat, including accompaniments) ☑

WARM-UP

March on spot with shoulder rolls

Stand tall and march on the spot for a total of 2 minutes. For every 4 steps,
do a full shoulder roll, pulling shoulders forward, up, back and down.

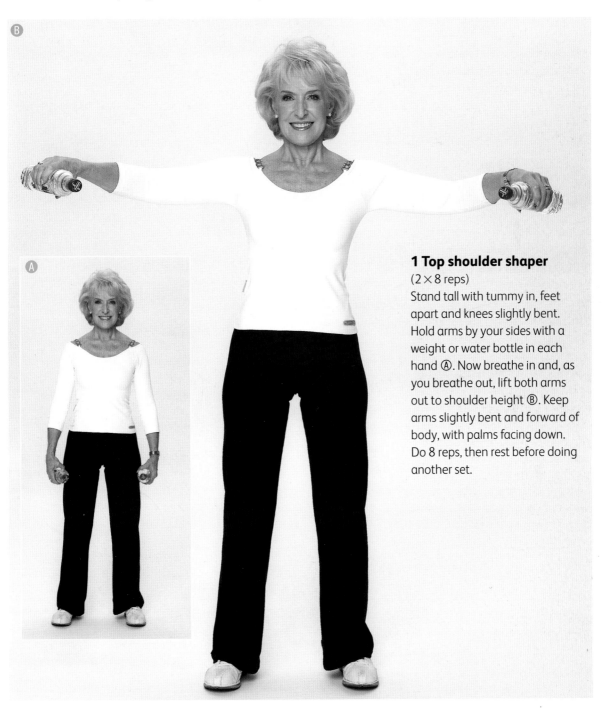

1 Top shoulder shaper

(2 × 8 reps)

Stand tall with tummy in, feet apart and knees slightly bent. Hold arms by your sides with a weight or water bottle in each hand Ⓐ. Now breathe in and, as you breathe out, lift both arms out to shoulder height Ⓑ. Keep arms slightly bent and forward of body, with palms facing down. Do 8 reps, then rest before doing another set.

2 Tummy curl ▷

(3 × 10 reps)

Lie on back with both hands behind head, knees bent and feet hip width apart Ⓐ. Now breathe in and, as you breathe out, lift head and shoulders off floor, pulling your navel in towards spine Ⓑ. Keep your chin off your chest and look forward as you lift. Do 10 reps, then rest before doing another 2 sets.

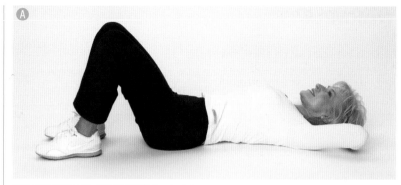

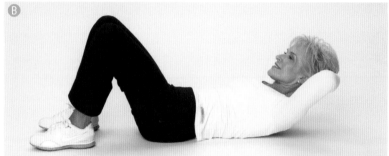

3 Bottom and inner thigh ▷ toner

(2 × 10 reps)

Still lying on back with knees bent, place a small, thick cushion between your knees Ⓐ. Make sure your feet are parallel and firmly planted on the floor. Now breathe in and, as you breathe out, squeeze cushion with your inner thighs and at the same time lift your bottom off floor without arching your back Ⓑ. Breathe in as you lower under control. Do 10 reps, then rest before doing another set.

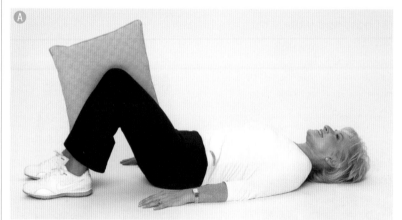

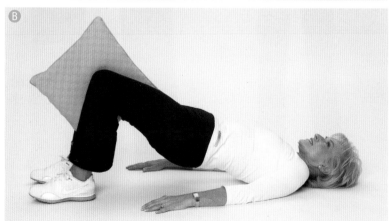

4 Spine strengthener ▶

(2 × 8 reps)

Lie on front with both elbows close to waist and palms facing up Ⓐ. Breathe in and, as you breathe out, lift head and shoulders just off the floor with head still facing floor Ⓑ. Pause for 2 seconds, then release. Do 8 reps, then rest before doing another set.

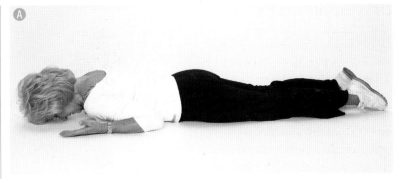

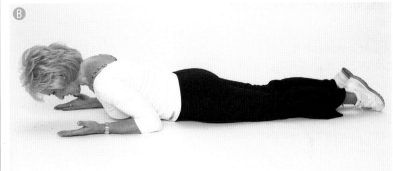

5 Chest and underarm toner ▶

(2 × 6 reps)

Come up onto your hands and knees with wrists in line with shoulders and your knees directly under hips Ⓐ. Pull tummy in to support your back, then breathe in as you bend elbows and take your forehead towards floor Ⓑ. Breathe out as you lift again without locking elbows at the top. Do 6 reps, then rest before doing another set.

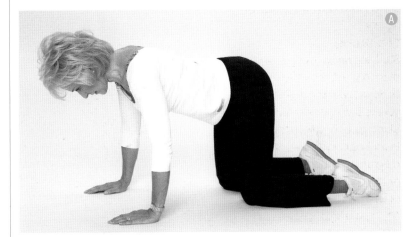

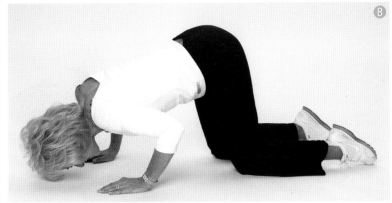

POST-WORKOUT STRETCHES

1 Tummy stretch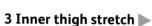

Lie on front with arms bent and elbows under shoulders. Keeping hips in contact with floor, lift chin forward slightly to feel a stretch in your tummy. Hold for 10 seconds, then release.

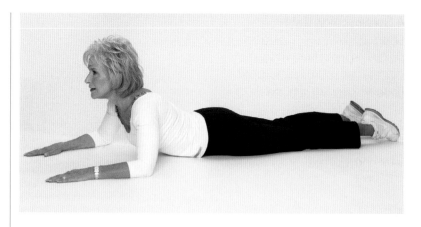

2 Back stretch ▶

Come up onto hands and knees and, as you pull your tummy in, arch your spine up towards the ceiling, letting your head drop down. Hold for 10 seconds, then release.

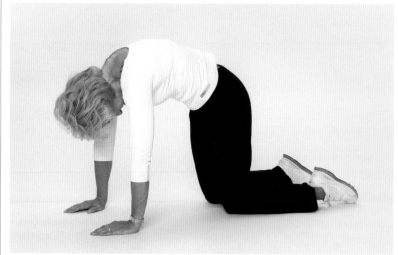

3 Inner thigh stretch ▶

Sit upright with soles of feet together and elbows resting on inside of thighs. Keeping your head up and back straight, lean forward and press elbows onto thighs. Hold for 10 seconds, then breathe in and, as you breathe out, press down further on thighs and hold for another 10 seconds.

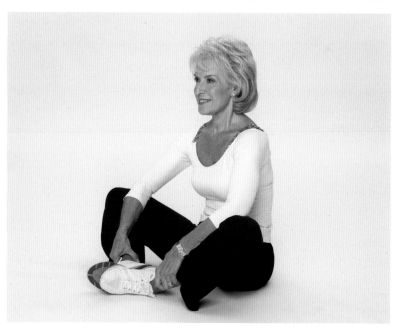

4 Underarm stretch ▶

Sit upright with legs crossed and place right hand behind right shoulder. Press left hand on right underarm to push right hand further down your back. Keep your head up and look straight ahead. Hold for 10 seconds, then change arms and repeat.

5 Chest stretch ▼

Place both hands behind you on floor. Draw shoulders back to feel a stretch across your chest, and hold for 10 seconds.

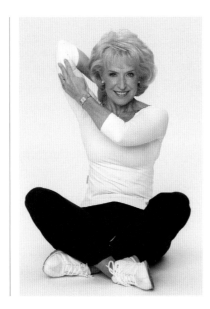

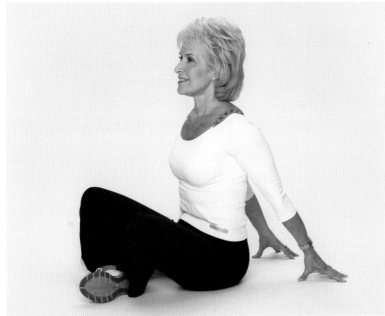

Exercise tip

It is really important to warm up before exercising as this helps to increase circulation and prevent injury and muscle soreness later. Although it's tempting to get going with the fat-burning exercises straight away, you will burn fat more efficiently if you have warmed up your muscles first. Remember, we burn fat in our muscles, so it makes sense to get your muscles (with their little engines called mitochondria) firing on all cylinders by the time you come to the fat-burning exercises in the aerobic section.

MOTIVATIONAL THOUGHT FOR THE DAY

Here are five tips to keep you on track this week.

1 Use your Portion Pots® or weigh out your daily portions of cereal, rice and pasta, etc., to ensure you stay within your calorie limit.

2 Remove the skin and fat from any poultry or meat before you put it on your plate, or before cooking if appropriate.

3 Avoid spreading butter, margarine or spread on your bread, as this adds loads of unnecessary calories. Instead, use low-fat sauces such as tomato ketchup, HP Fruity Sauce or very low-fat mayonnaise.

4 Dry-fry foods in a non-stick frying pan or wok. You can prepare many delicious low-fat dishes this way (e.g. stir-fries, curries, soups), and add any liquid or cooking sauces later, depending on the recipe.

5 Have a long drink before you start eating to help fill you up. Only cook the amount of food you need and serve it on a slightly smaller dinner plate than usual so that it looks like a generous serving size. This avoids waste and the temptation to go for second helpings.

Day 9

Now that you're into the swing of things for week two of the 14-Day Fast Track you are probably feeling quite excited. You are already past the halfway stage of this really strict couple of weeks and your body is getting used to eating healthier – and less – food than before. You are sleeping better, you wake up more rested and are feeling fitter. You have to be, as you are exercising regularly, your muscles are working harder and the aerobic exercise will have made your heart and lungs more efficient. Well done and keep up the good work!

Today's toning exercises, which are done with the help of a chair, will work your waist, stomach, outer and front thighs and your shoulders.

MENU

Breakfast
- 1 Weetabix or Shredded Wheat served with milk from allowance plus 1 tsp sugar and 1 thinly sliced medium banana ☑

Mid-morning power snack
- 1 medium pear ☑

Lunch
- 1 Batchelors Cup a Soup. Plus 1 Müllerlight yogurt (max. 150 kcal) and 1 kiwi fruit

OR
- 1 × 175g oven-baked sweet potato topped with 75g baked beans, served with a side salad tossed in fat-free dressing of your choice ☑

Mid-afternoon power snack
- 1 blue Portion Pot® (75g) tomato salsa served with 1 carrot, 1 celery stick and 1 × 5cm piece cucumber, all sliced into crudités ☑

Dinner
- Cheesy Quorn Bake: Dry-fry 1 finely chopped red onion and 1 crushed garlic clove in a non-stick pan until soft, then stir in 100g Quorn mince and cook for a further 2 minutes. Add 200g chopped tomatoes, 250g tomato passata, ½–1 tsp vegetable stock powder, ½ tbsp chives and reduce to a gentle simmer. While the Quorn mixture is simmering, heat a non-stick griddle pan and cook 150g chopped courgettes on both sides until lightly browned, seasoning with black pepper. Layer the courgettes and Quorn mixture in an ovenproof dish. Pour 150g 2% fat Greek yogurt over the top and add 25g grated Rosemary Conley low-fat Mature Cheese (or vegetarian alternative) and black pepper to taste. Bake in a preheated oven at 200C, 400F, Gas Mark 6 for 20 minutes until the cheese has melted and the dish is hot all the way through. Garnish with chopped chives ☑ P

OR
- Lamb and Mushroom Goulash (see recipe, p.215) served with green vegetables

WARM-UP

Ski swings

Stand tall and lift both arms overhead, pulling your tummy in. Now swing arms down and past thighs as you bend knees and hips. Keep your back straight and keep looking forward. Come up again and repeat ski swings for 1 minute.

FIVE-MINUTE TONE-UP

1 Seated side bend ▶

(3 × 10 reps alternate sides)
Sit on front third of chair seat, holding a weight or water bottle in each hand. Pull tummy in very tight and bend to one side without dropping forward or back, then come back to centre and bend to other side. Do 10 reps (5 each side), keeping it slow and controlled, then rest before doing another 2 sets.

2 Posture improver ▶

(2 × 10 reps)
Sit upright with a weight or water bottle in each hand and each arm bent at 90 degrees as if you were holding a large tray Ⓐ. Keeping elbows close to waist, pull hands further apart Ⓐ and pull shoulders down to feel shoulder blades working. Return to start position and do 10 reps slowly, then rest before doing another set.

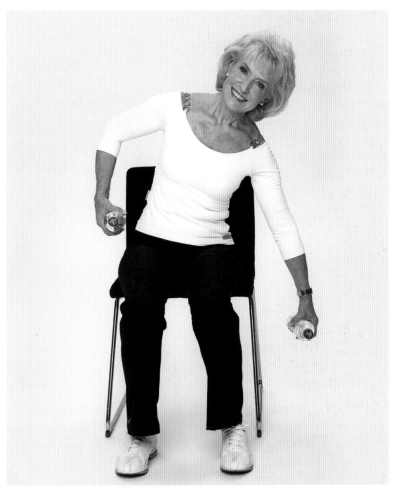

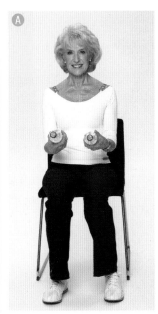

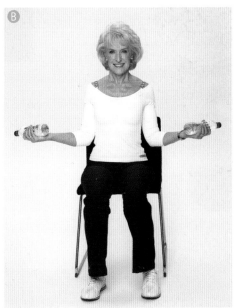

3 Thigh shaper ▶

(2 × 10 reps)

Stand and hold on to back of chair with feet parallel and hip width apart. Now push hips back, bending knees in line with ankles and with most of your body weight in heels (you should be able to wiggle your toes!). Come up slowly without locking knees at the top. Do 10 reps, then rest before doing another set.

4 Outer thigh toner ▼

(2 × 8 reps each leg)

Lift left leg out to side with foot flexed, keeping leg straight, trunk upright and tummy in. Lower again and keep lifting same leg for 8 reps, then change legs and repeat. Rest before doing another set.

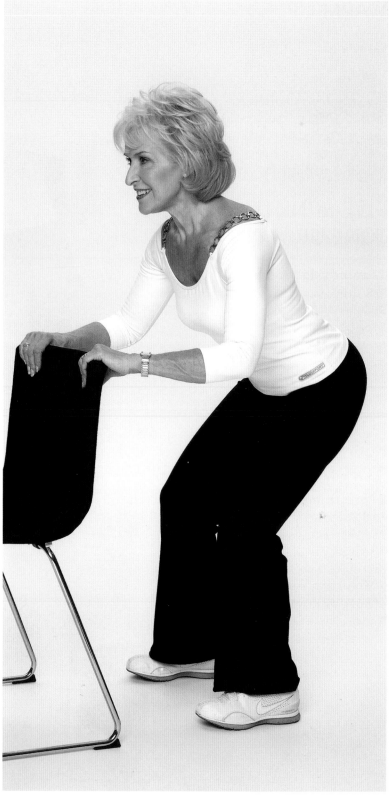

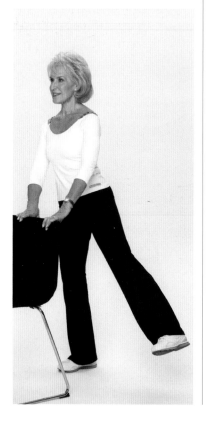

5 Tummy curl ▶

(2 × 10 reps)

Lie on back with lower legs supported on chair seat and both hands behind head Ⓐ. Pull your tummy in very tight, then breathe in and, as you breathe out, lift head and shoulders off floor and keep looking forward Ⓑ. Lower again under control with tummy still held in. Do 10 reps, then rest before doing another set.

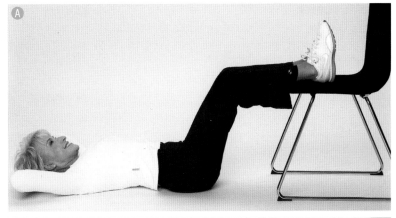

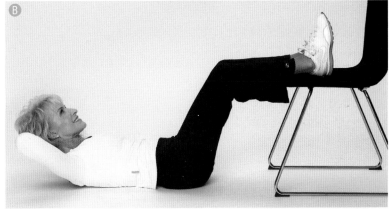

POST-WORKOUT STRETCHES

1 Upper back stretch ▶

Sit on front third of chair seat, bring both arms forward at chest height and drop head down. Press arms forward and shoulder blades back to feel a stretch across upper back. Hold for 10 seconds, then release.

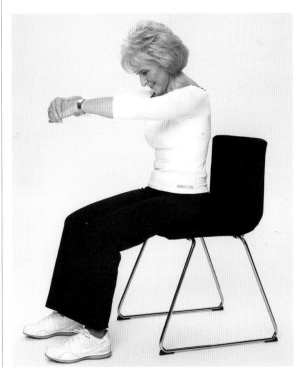

2 Waist stretch ▼

Place right hand on chair seat for support and lift left arm. Keeping both hips firmly on chair seat, bend to right without leaning forward or back, to feel a stretch down your left side. Hold stretch for 10 seconds, then change sides and repeat.

3 Outer thigh and hip stretch ▼

Bring one ankle onto opposite knee and, holding chair seat for support, let the knee drop outwards to feel a stretch in the outer thigh and hip. (If this is too difficult, just cross legs.) Hold stretch for 10 seconds, then change legs and repeat.

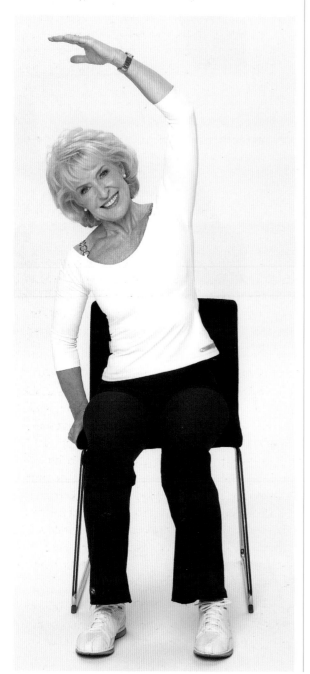

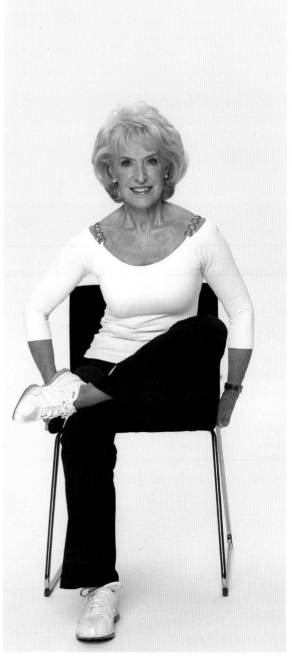

4 Front thigh stretch ▼

Stand and hold on to back of chair with right hand. Take left ankle in left hand (or hold your trouser leg or sock) and bring knees in line with each other. Press your hip forward to feel a stretch down the front of your thigh. Hold for 10 seconds, then change legs and repeat.

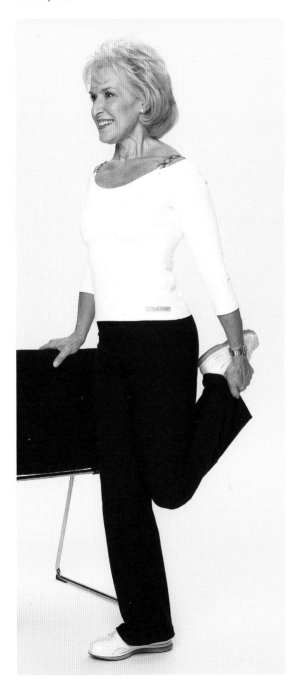

AEROBIC CHALLENGE

Go for a brisk walk or swim or a bike ride for 30 minutes.

Exercise tip

Yesterday I talked about the importance of warming up before exercise. Today, I want to emphasise the vital role of cooling down and stretching after your workout. During a workout, you are challenging your muscles and this can produce a build up of lactic acid and cause your muscles to ache later – sometimes two days later. Stretching the muscles you've used in your workout will help to eliminate this discomfort. In the daily plans in this book, I have included the appropriate stretches for each day and you only need to hold each one for 10 seconds.

MOTIVATIONAL THOUGHT FOR THE DAY

Does your stomach feel flatter this morning and your clothes looser? Soon you will need to buy some new clothes. I did hear of one slimmer 'hanging on' for as long as possible before buying a smaller size only to have their trousers fall down one day as they walked down the street!

Rather than investing in new clothes that are only going to fit you for a short while, why not have a look in a charity shop or dress agency for something nice to wear temporarily. I always take my clothes to one of these outlets when I'm bored with them or I've had second thoughts after buying them and felt that, after all, they didn't do a lot for me. Sometimes brand new, or at least nearly-new clothes, can be found in charity shops and there are real bargains to be had. And when you drop down to the next dress size, you can take the first lot back and buy some new, smaller ones. I suggest you only invest in new clothes when you reach your ultimate goal.

One important thing, though. Make sure you keep at least one – your largest – garment as a reminder of how big you once were, as you will forget later when you get used to being slim.

Day 10

Ten days into the 14-Day Fast Track diet and you may be feeling peckish. I have tried to select low-Gi foods to keep your blood glucose levels stable and help you feel fuller for longer. Be sure to eat your power snacks and drink plenty of fluids. Often hunger can be confused with dehydration, so keep well hydrated.

When I trialled this low-Gi diet I was surprised at how well the women and men who followed it coped with the very restricted calorie allowance in the first two weeks. They all said they hardly felt hungry during that time and were amazed at how much healthier they felt in such a short time. The feelings of general wellbeing they reported were significant. So stick with the diet and do the exercises every day and soon you will feel like a new person too.

Today is an aerobic day so there are no toning exercises. Do make sure you find time to do your fat-burning aerobics, though, to help speed up your weight loss.

MENU

Breakfast
- ½ fresh grapefruit plus 1 medium-sized poached egg served on 1 small slice toasted wholegrain bread spread with Marmite ☑

Mid-morning power snack
- 1 yellow Portion Pot® (125ml) apple juice ☑

Lunch
- 100g cooked chicken breast (no skin), sliced, and served with a large mixed salad and 1 tbsp Hellmann's Extra Light Mayonnaise **P**
OR
- Stir-Fried Rice Noodles (see recipe, p.221) served with salad ☑

Mid-afternoon power snack
- 75g sliced mango ☑

Dinner
- 1 × 150g (raw weight) lean pork steak (all fat removed), grilled, served with 115g boiled new potatoes (with skins), 200g other vegetables of your choice, plus low-fat gravy and 1 tbsp apple sauce
OR
- 1 × 300g pack Rosemary Conley Solo Slim Spicy Vegetable and Lentil Dahl (order from www.rosemaryconley.com). Plus 1 low-fat yogurt (max. 150 kcal and 5 % fat) ☑

WARM-UP

Stair step-ups

Using a single step (such as the bottom step of your stairs or your front doorstep), step up and down for 2 minutes. Lead with the right leg for 1 minute, then pause and change to lead with the left leg. Make sure the whole foot makes contact on each step.

AEROBIC CHALLENGE

Do 40 minutes of aerobic work, choosing one of the following activities: working out to a fitness DVD or at an aerobics class, swimming, cycling, brisk walking or using cardio equipment at the gym (e.g. stepper, treadmill, cross-trainer, exercise bike).

POST-AEROBIC STRETCHES

1 Calf stretch ▼

Place one foot in front of the other, with both feet pointing forward (hold on to a wall or sturdy surface for support if you wish). Bend front knee in line with ankle and keep back leg straight with heel pressing down. Lean further forward to feel a stretch in calf of back leg and hold for 10 seconds. Do the lower calf stretch (exercise 2, p.78) before changing legs.

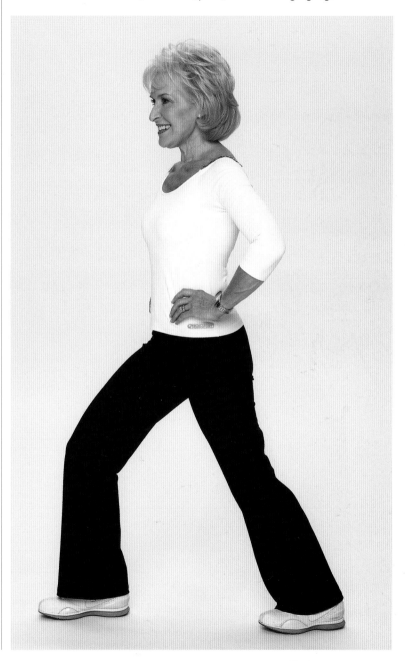

2 Lower calf stretch ▼

Bring your back foot half a step in and bend both knees with feet still pointing forward. Keep both heels on floor and your body upright as you look straight ahead and hold for 10 seconds. Change legs and repeat both calf stretches.

3 Back thigh stretch ▼

Straighten your front leg and keep your back leg bent. With spine straight, lean forward slightly to feel a stretch in back thigh of straight leg. Hold for 10 seconds, then change legs and repeat.

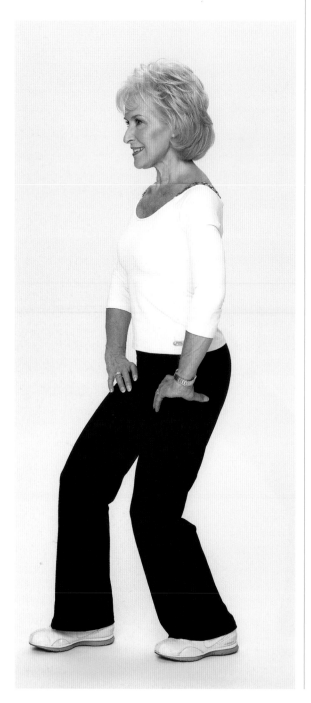

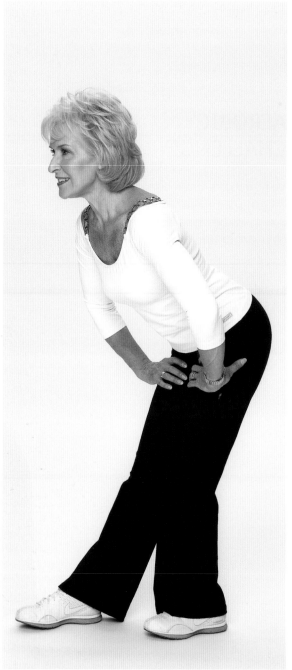

4 Front of hip stretch ▶

Bend front leg and lift heel of back foot. With your weight equally distributed between both legs, trunk upright and tummy in, press pelvis forward to feel a stretch at top of hip. Hold for 10 seconds, then change legs and repeat.

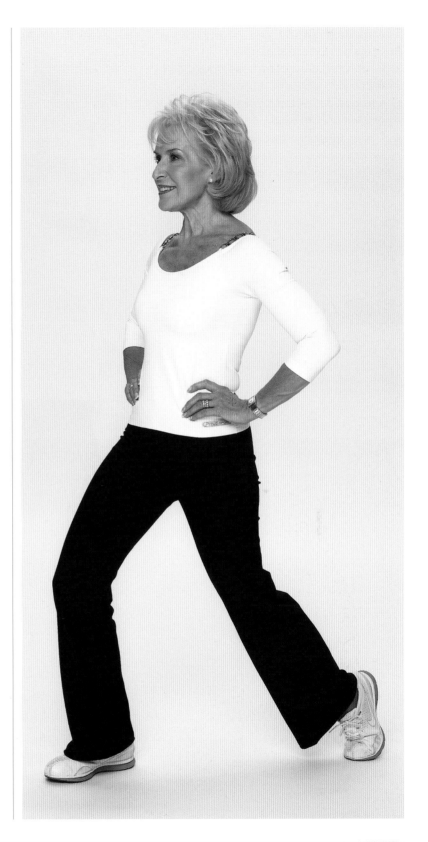

5 Front thigh stretch ▶

Stand upright and take hold of one ankle with hand (place other hand on wall or back of chair for support if necessary). Bring knees in line with each other and keep supporting leg slightly bent. Gently push hip of raised leg forward to stretch front of thigh. Hold stretch for 10 seconds, then change legs and repeat.

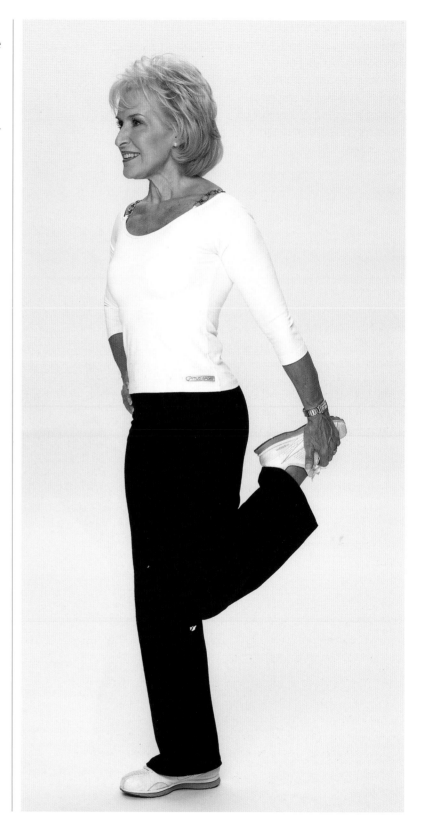

6 Inner thigh stretch ▶

Stand tall and take legs out wide. Bend one knee in line with ankle, keeping other leg straight with foot pointing forward, to feel a stretch in inner thigh of straight leg. Hold for 10 seconds, then change legs and repeat.

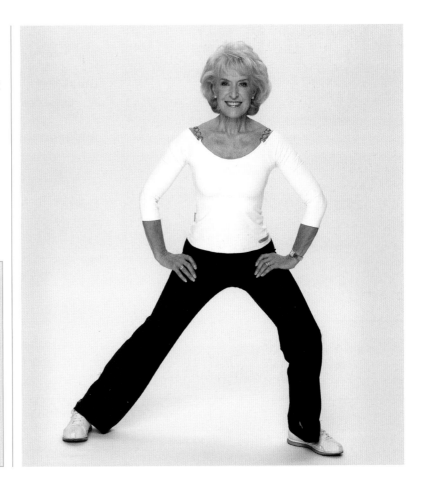

Exercise tip

When we do aerobic exercise, the fat-burning takes place in our muscles. The stronger our muscles, the more fat we burn, so it's important to make the effort to keep our muscles strong. Using a toning band or light handweights is a great way to increase the intensity of a toning workout.

MOTIVATIONAL THOUGHT FOR THE DAY

When we lose weight and burn body fat it's important to look after our skin so that it 'shrinks' with us and doesn't end up being saggy. There will be some natural shrinkage and then, when we exercise, the extra blood pumping around the body close to the skin's surface warms the skin, making it more metabolically active and more toned. It works like magic in helping our skin to firm up.

When I meet slimmers who have lost massive amounts of weight – 10 stone is not uncommon – I always ask about their skincare routine. They tell me that they moisturise and massage their skin every morning after showering and this, combined with all the exercise they did to achieve their amazing weight loss, had a remarkable effect on their skin.

In 2008 I decided to ask a manufacturer if they could develop an inexpensive body toning and moisturising body cream that would be effective at helping skin to shrink back on a weight loss plan. I told them I wouldn't put my name to it unless it was proven to work. A cream was developed, put through a clinical trial and launched later that year. It has proved extremely popular with readers and members of our clubs alike and the feedback has been very positive (see www.rosemaryconley.com for further information).

But, remember, any body lotion massaged into your skin is better than none and will have some effect in helping your skin to contract and stay healthy.

Day 11

I hope your encourager is supporting you and that you are sharing your thoughts and feelings with them. And how are you getting on talking to yourself as a third party? Are you saying positive and encouraging things to yourself and affirming your progress to date? You didn't become overweight overnight and you won't get slim overnight either, so be patient and think forward, upward and onward.

Remember, you can choose meals from anywhere in this book as long as you substitute a lunch for a lunch or a dinner for a dinner. It doesn't matter which one you select. The important thing is that you enjoy what you are eating.

In today's exercise programme I've focused on the abdominals, backside, inner and front thighs, and the chest and underarms. Practise these exercises regularly and you will see a significant difference in your muscle strength and your overall body shape.

MENU

Breakfast
- 2 large bananas ☑

Mid-morning power snack
- 1 yellow Portion Pot® (125ml) fresh orange juice ☑

Lunch
- Spread 2 slices wholegrain bread spread with HP Fruity Sauce (or similar) and make into a sandwich with 3 grilled turkey rashers, then toast in a sandwich toaster or double-sided electric grill
OR
- Garlic Mushroom Pasta (see recipe, p.219) ☑

Mid-afternoon power snack
- 2 satsumas ☑

Dinner
- Spicy Pork Steak: Mix together 1 tsp ground cumin, 1 tsp ground ginger and 1 tsp smoked paprika on a plate, then press 300g lean pork steak into the spices and season with salt and pepper. Cook the steak in a health grill for 8–10 minutes or under a conventional grill for 8–10 minutes each side. Serve hot with a mixed salad or vegetables of your choice 🄿
OR
- Vegetable Chilli: Dry-fry 1 chopped onion in a preheated non-stick pan. Add 1 × 200g can mixed beans in chilli sauce and 1 × 200g can chopped tomatoes plus chopped vegetables (e.g. courgettes, mushrooms, carrots, peppers) and simmer for 15–20 minutes. Serve with 1 blue Portion Pot® (55g uncooked weight) or 1 red Portion Pot® (144g cooked weight) basmati rice ☑

WARM-UP

March on spot with tummy pull-ins

Stand tall and march on the spot, letting the arms swing naturally. Every 10 steps, really pull your tummy in tight and then relax it for 10 steps.

FIVE-MINUTE TONE-UP

1 Standing squat

(2 × 12 reps)

Stand tall with feet parallel and hip width apart. Hold a weight or water bottle in each hand at side of thighs Ⓐ. Bend your hips back as if about to sit in a chair, keeping knees in line with ankles and most of your body weight in heels Ⓑ. Push up slowly again without locking knees at top. Do 12 reps, then rest before doing another set.

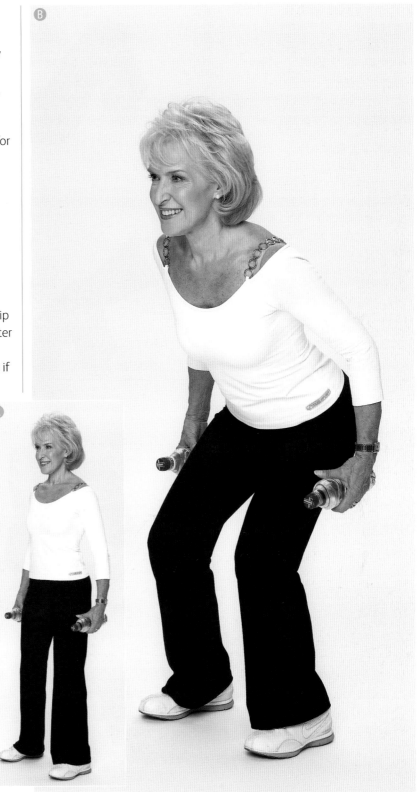

2 Tummy curl with ▶ leg raise

(2 × 8 reps alternate legs)
Lie on your back with knees bent, feet together and tummy in, and place both hands behind head with elbows raised slightly Ⓐ. Breathe in and, as you breathe out, lift head and shoulders off floor and at same time extend right leg, keeping knees firmly together Ⓑ. Breathe in as you slowly lower head and leg, holding tummy in. Repeat, raising other leg, and keep changing legs. Do 8 reps (4 each leg), then rest before doing another set.

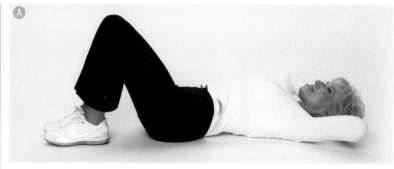

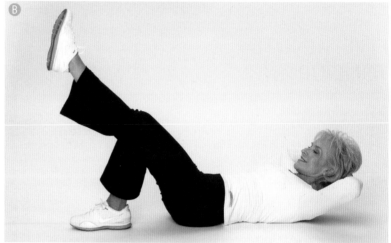

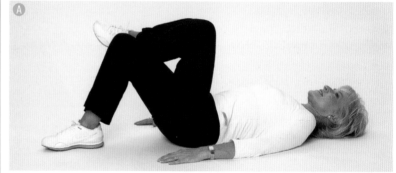

3 One side hip lift ▶

(2 × 6 reps each leg)
Place arms by sides and rest one ankle on opposite knee. Bring heel of other foot a little closer to hips Ⓐ. Breathe in and, as you breathe out, lift hips off floor without arching your back Ⓑ. Lower again slowly and do 6 reps on same side, then change legs and repeat. Rest before doing another set.

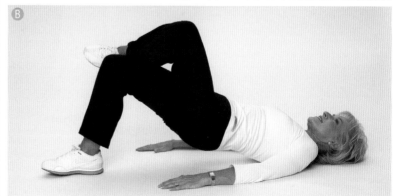

4 Inner thigh toner ▷

(2 × 12 reps each leg)

Lie on side, propped up on your elbow, with top leg bent over bottom leg and top knee resting on a rolled towel. Straighten your bottom leg and pull your tummy in to keep your trunk still Ⓐ. Now lift and lower the bottom leg under control 12 times Ⓑ, then rest before doing another set. Roll over to change legs and repeat on the other side.

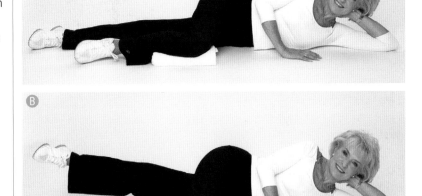

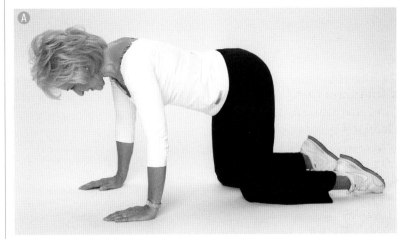

5 Chest and underarm ▷ toner

(2 × 8 reps)

Come up onto your hands and knees with wrists in line with shoulders and your knees directly under hips Ⓐ. Pull your tummy in to support your back, then breathe in as you bend elbows and take forehead towards floor Ⓑ. Breathe out as you lift again without locking elbows at top. Do 8 reps, then rest before doing another set.

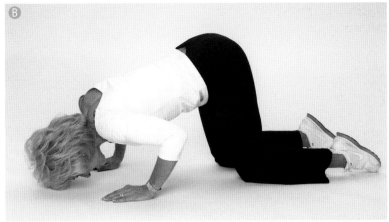

POST-WORKOUT STRETCHES

1 Tummy stretch ▼

Lie on front with arms at sides and elbows bent. Now prop up on your elbows, keeping hips in contact with floor, and lift chin forward slightly to feel a stretch in your tummy. Hold for 10 seconds, then release.

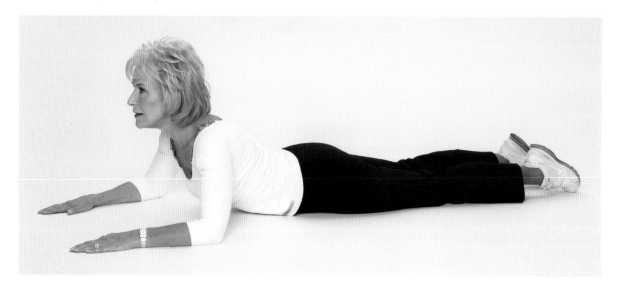

2 Front thigh stretch ▼

Lie on front, bend one knee and take hold of foot with hand on same side (or hold on to your trouser leg or sock). Relax your upper body and gently press your hip into floor to feel a stretch down front of thigh. Hold for 10 seconds, then change legs and repeat.

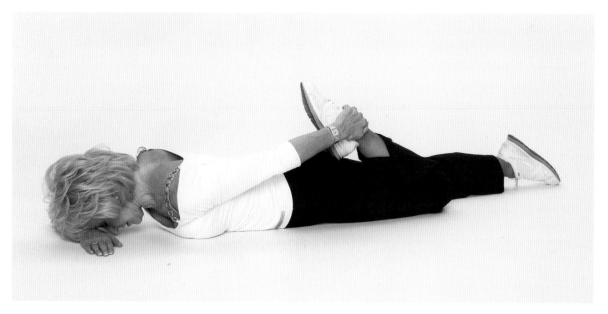

3 Underarm stretch ▶

Sit upright with legs crossed and place right hand behind right shoulder. Press left hand on right underarm to push right hand further down your back. Keep head up and look straight ahead. Hold for 10 seconds, then change arms and repeat.

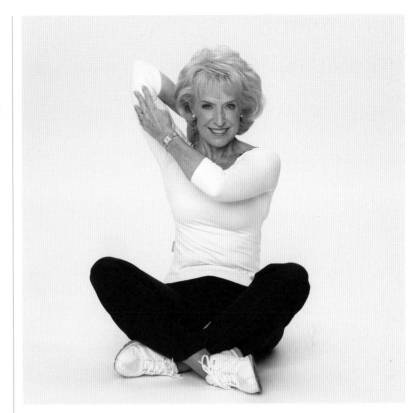

4 Chest stretch ▶

Sit upright and place both hands behind you on floor. Draw shoulders back to feel a stretch across chest. Hold for 10 seconds, then release.

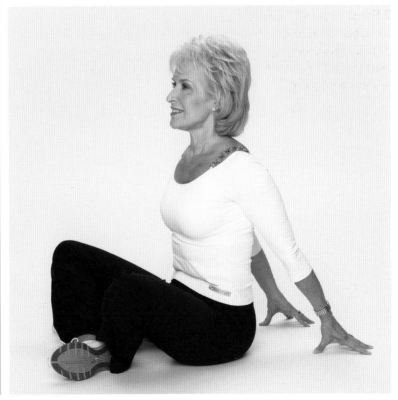

5 Inner thigh stretch ▶

Sit upright with soles of feet together and elbows resting on inside of thighs. Keeping your head up and back straight, lean forward and press elbows onto thighs. Hold for 10 seconds, then breathe in and, as you breathe out, press down further on thighs and hold for another 10 seconds.

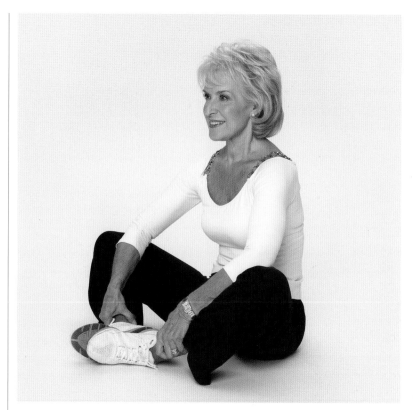

6 Back thigh stretch ▶

Sit upright with one leg straight out in front and the other bent. Place hands on floor at either side of straight leg and lean forward from the hips to feel a stretch in back of thigh. Hold for 10 seconds, then try to lean a little further forward for another 10 seconds. Change legs and repeat.

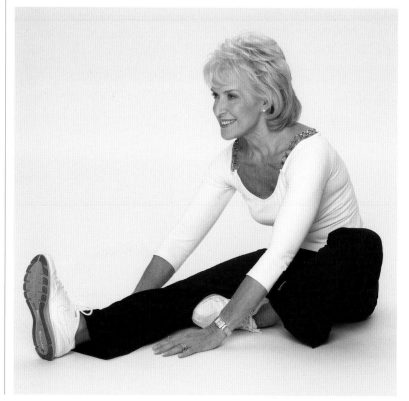

AEROBIC CHALLENGE

Walk up and down stairs 4 times consecutively and repeat 4 times during the day.

Exercise tip

If you want a flat stomach, you need to do plenty of toning exercises such as stomach crunches and ab curls in order to strengthen your abdominals. However, these exercises in themselves will not get rid of the fat, but when you do your aerobic exercise, your stronger abdominal muscles will encourage fat burning from around the whole body much more efficiently and that includes the abdominal area.

MOTIVATIONAL THOUGHT FOR THE DAY

I am a firm believer in only weighing and measuring ourselves once a week however tempting it might be to pop on the scales midweek. The problem is that fluctuating body fluid levels and all manner of other factors can affect our weight. If you were to weigh yourself now, you might find you've made great progress but then see little difference between now and your weigh-in session on Day 15, and you will only be disheartened. So please be patient and wait until the 'official' weigh-in day – and then you can celebrate!

Scales should be placed on a flat, non-carpeted surface for greatest accuracy, but keep them out of the bathroom. Bathrooms are damp and steamy and this can affect the mechanism in the scales. Body fat monitors are very popular now and are an easy way to see how much body fat you have lost. However, only check your body fat reading monthly or, better still, bi-monthly as, again, the reading can vary, depending on your body's fluid levels, and an occasional reading is likely to be more significant and encouraging. Do not use a body fat monitor if you are pregnant or have a pacemaker fitted, as body fat monitors work by passing a tiny electric current through the body. Fat acts as an electrical insulator, while muscle conducts the current very efficiently. The voltage drop across the body therefore depends on the relative amounts of fat and muscle.

Measuring the different areas of your body is important too, because when we are exercising regularly we sometimes lose inches without losing weight. All that matters is that we are getting smaller.

Day 12

Only three days to go before the end of this 14-Day Fast Track! The feeling of satisfaction and achievement when you reach Day 15 will be amazing. From then on, you will have the opportunity to enjoy treats, alcohol and puddings! But for now, you must concentrate on this last run on the homeward straight. Stay focused, exercise loads, drink plenty of water or low-cal drinks and DON'T CHEAT!

Today's toning exercises focus on the waist and stomach area, the inner and outer thighs, and the shoulders.

MENU

Breakfast
- 1 Quorn bacon-style rasher, grilled, served with 1 yellow Portion Pot® (115g) baked beans plus 1 tomato, halved and grilled, and 50g grilled mushrooms V P

Mid-morning power snack
- 2 kiwi fruit V

Lunch
- Prawn Wrap: Spread 1 tortilla wrap with 1 tsp Thai sweet chilli dipping sauce, then fill with 50g cooked prawns, chopped salad leaves, peppers, cucumber, celery and cherry tomatoes and wrap into a parcel before cutting in half horizontally to make 2 wraps
OR
- Large salad of grated carrots, beansprouts, chopped peppers, celery, tomatoes, cucumber and red onion, served with 1 blue Portion Pot® (100g) low-fat cottage cheese, plus 1 tbsp Hellmann's Extra Light Mayonnaise; followed by 1 low-fat yogurt (max. 100 kcal and 5% fat) V

Mid-afternoon power snack
- 1 small bowl of mixed salad tossed in fat-free dressing V

Dinner
- Lamb Stir-Fry: Cut 150g lean lamb steak into strips and dry-fry with ½ chopped onion and ½ crushed garlic clove in a non-stick pan over a high heat for 1–2 minutes. Add 1 tsp mint sauce, 75g stir-fry vegetables and ½ tbsp soy sauce and toss well before cooking for 7–8 minutes. Serve on a bed of lightly cooked beansprouts P
OR
- 2 Quorn sausages, grilled, served with ½ pack readymade cauliflower cheese (max. 200 kcal and 5% fat) and green vegetables of your choice V

WARM-UP

Knee lifts with pull-downs

Stand upright with hands high and tummy pulled in. Lift alternate knees and as you lift each knee, pull arms down to either side of knees. Keep your tummy in and your back straight and continue for 1 minute.

2 Tummy curl with ▶ leg raise

(2 × 10 reps alternate legs)
Bring feet and knees together and place both hands behind head with elbows raised slightly Ⓐ. Pull your tummy in, then breathe in and, as you breathe out, lift head and shoulders off floor and at same time extend right leg, keeping knees firmly together Ⓑ. Breathe in as you slowly lower head and leg, holding your tummy in. Repeat, raising other leg, and keep changing legs. Do 10 reps (5 each leg), then rest before doing another set.

FIVE-MINUTE TONE-UP

1 Waist shaper (2 × 10 reps alternate sides) ▼

Lie on back with knees bent, feet flat on floor and hip width apart. Place hands behind head and pull tummy in tight, then breathe in and, as you breathe out, lift right shoulder and left knee at same time, aiming shoulder towards knee. Keep your chin off chest and keep hips on floor. Lower again, then repeat to other side. Do 10 reps, changing sides each time, then rest before doing another set.

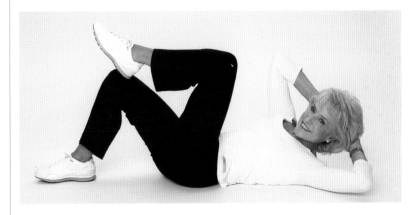

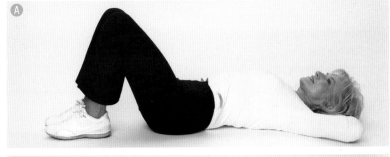

Ⓐ

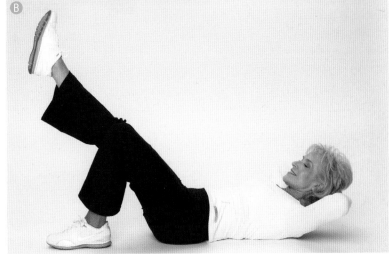

Ⓑ

3 Outer thigh shaper ▶

(2 × 16 reps each leg)

Lie on side, bend bottom leg up to 90 degrees and push top leg out straight in line with hip, with foot flexed. Hold a weight or water bottle on thigh Ⓐ. Pull tummy in to hold trunk still, then lift top leg under control Ⓑ and slowly lower again. Do 16 reps on this leg, then roll over and repeat with other leg. Rest before doing another set.

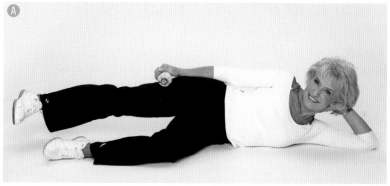

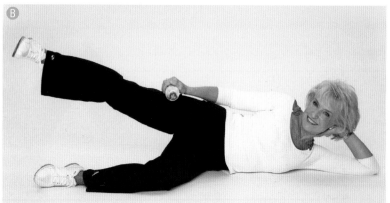

4 Inner thigh toner ▶

(2 × 16 reps each leg)

Lie on side, propped up on your elbow, with top leg bent over bottom leg and top knee resting on a rolled towel. Straighten your bottom leg and keep it off floor slightly Ⓐ. Pull your tummy in to keep your trunk still, then lift bottom leg under control Ⓑ and lower again. Do 16 reps, then rest before doing another set. Roll over to change legs and repeat on other side.

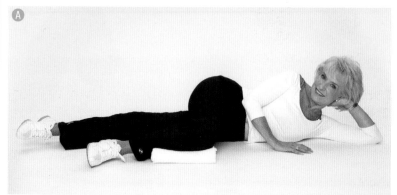

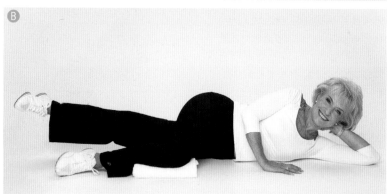

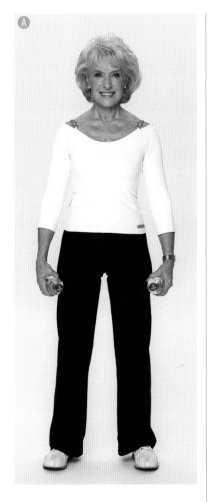

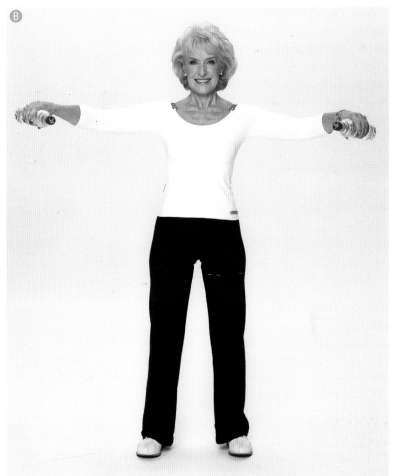

5 Top shoulder shaper ▲
(2 × 8 reps)

Stand tall with tummy pulled in, feet apart and knees slightly bent, with arms by your sides and a weight or water bottle in each hand Ⓐ. Now lift both arms out to sides at shoulder height Ⓑ. Keep arms slightly bent and in front of body with palms facing down. Do 8 reps, then rest before doing another set.

POST-WORKOUT STRETCHES

1 Shoulder stretch ▶

Sit upright with legs crossed and bring right arm across trunk at shoulder height. Use other arm to gently press on upper arm to stretch outside of shoulder. Hold for 10 seconds, then change arms and repeat.

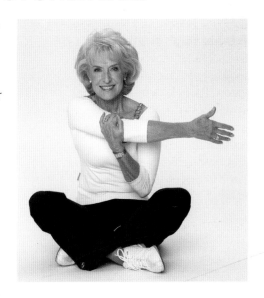

2 Waist stretch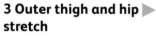

Still sitting up tall with legs crossed, lift right arm and lean over to left side, keeping both hips on floor and without leaning forward or back. Hold for 10 seconds, then change sides and repeat.

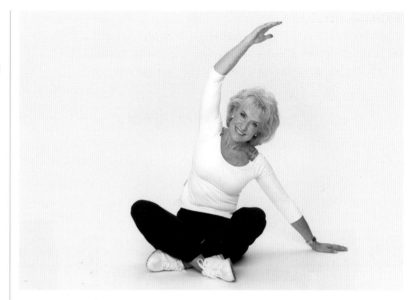

3 Outer thigh and hip stretch

Sit upright with legs straight out in front and bring left foot over right leg, placing foot flat on floor. Place left hand on floor for support and right hand across left knee. Use pressure of right arm to pull left leg further across body to feel a stretch in outer thigh and hip. Hold for 10 seconds, then change legs and repeat.

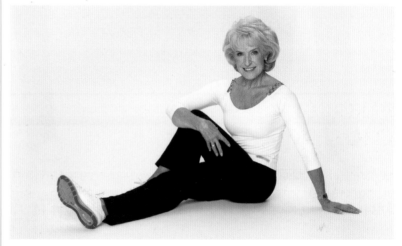

4 Inner thigh stretch

Sit upright with soles of feet together and elbows resting on inside of thighs. Keeping your head up and back straight, lean forward and press elbows onto thighs. Hold for 10 seconds, then breathe in and, as you breathe out, press down further on thighs and hold for another 10 seconds.

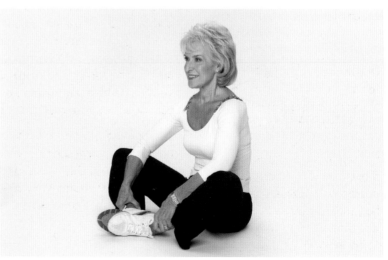

5 Tummy stretch ▼

Lie on front with arms bent at sides. Now prop yourself up on elbows, keeping hips in contact with floor, and lift chin forward slightly to feel a stretch in your tummy. Hold for 10 seconds, then release.

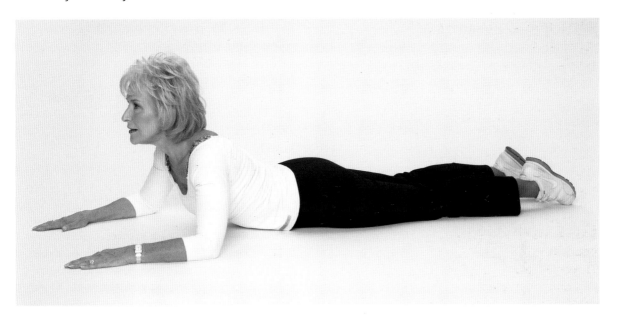

AEROBIC CHALLENGE

Go for a brisk 30-minute walk and aim to clock up at least 10,000 steps on your pedometer. Alternatively, walk up and down stairs 5 times consecutively and repeat later in the day.

Exercise tip

One of the most effective ways to trim inches from your waist is to use a hula hoop or do a Salsacise workout. Moving the hips from side to side in a fast but small and controlled movement works the waist and abdominal muscles. I had never had such a small waist as when I was training for my first Salsacise DVD.

MOTIVATIONAL THOUGHT FOR THE DAY

Today would be a good day to flick through some fashion magazines or catalogues and think about what type of clothes you'd like to wear when you are slim. Slipping on a dress that is several sizes smaller than you used to wear will give you so much pleasure.

Would you consider yourself to be an 'apple' shape (large tummy and slim arms and legs), a 'heart' shape (large busted with slim legs and arms) or a 'pear' shape (small bust, narrow waist and large hips, thighs and arms)? It is helpful to recognise what type of shape you are and then dress accordingly. By making careful clothes choices you can address any imbalances you see in your figure, accentuating your good points and minimising the not so good ones.

Colours are really important too. Have you noticed that if someone tells you that a certain dress or top suits you, often it's the colour that has caught their eye. Learn which colours make you come alive and which ones don't. With a 'new you' in the making, it is worth using every ace in the pack to make sure you look your absolute best.

Day 13

For the next two days I am going to encourage you to step up your aerobic activity quite significantly. In addition to doing today's toning exercises, which focus on the waist, back, outer and front thighs and shoulders, I would like you to take every opportunity you can to be active. Walk up and down stairs whenever you have time, or go for an extra-brisk walk or jog. Be ultra-good with your food portion sizes and don't 'guesstimate'.

Try to stay busy so you don't get bored and start thinking about food! Avoid going food shopping for the next couple of days if you can – you might be tempted to buy something you'll regret.

MENU

Breakfast
■ 2 eggs scrambled with milk from allowance and served with 100g grilled tomatoes and unlimited grilled mushrooms ✓ P

Mid-morning power snack
■ 1 yellow Portion Pot® (70g) blueberries, topped with 1 tsp low-fat natural yogurt ✓

Lunch
■ Homemade Vegetable Soup (makes enough for approx. 6 servings): Bring 2 litres of water to the boil in a large pan, then add 2 vegetable stock cubes and 400g peeled and trimmed vegetables (e.g. carrots, parsnips, onion, cabbage) or leftover vegetables and boil until cooked. Remove from the heat, add some chopped coriander and black pepper and leave to cool a little. Pour the soup in small batches in a food processor and blend for a few seconds, then transfer to a storage container or jug and allow to cool before storing or freezing. Reheat as required, allowing 300ml per serving and accompany with a slice of toasted wholegrain bread ✓

Mid-afternoon power snack
■ 1 fat-free yogurt (max. 50 kcal) ✓

Dinner
■ Oven-Baked Salmon: Place 1 × 110g salmon steak in an ovenproof dish, top with 1 tsp Thai sweet chilli dipping sauce and the juice of $\frac{1}{2}$ lime. Bake in a preheated oven at 200C, 400F, Gas Mark 6 for 8–10 minutes, or until cooked. Serve with 100g boiled new potatoes (with skins) and unlimited green vegetables OR
■ Prawn (or Quorn) Saag (see recipe, p.217) served with 1 green Portion Pot (170g) cooked egg noodles or 1 blue Portion Pot® (55g uncooked weight) or 1 red Portion Pot® (144g cooked weight) basmati rice per person ✓
Plus 1 meringue nest topped with 2 tbsps 0% fat Greek yogurt and 2 sliced strawberries

WARM-UP

Pretend skipping

Imagine you are holding a skipping rope. Begin a small bounce on the spot as you pretend to turn the rope. You can turn around in a circle and even do some figure 8s.

FIVE-MINUTE TONE-UP

1 Waist shaper

(3 × 10 reps alternate sides)
Stand tall with tummy in tight, holding a weight or water bottle in

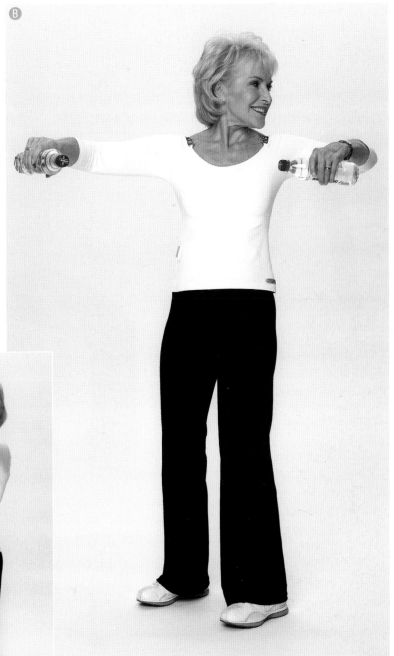

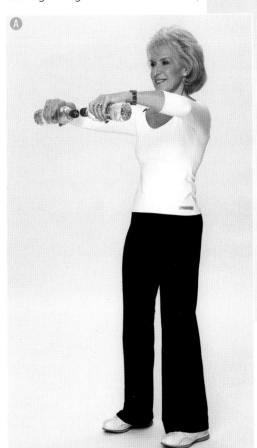

each hand, and bring both arms in front at shoulder height Ⓐ. Pull left elbow back, bending arm and keeping it at shoulder height with shoulders down and relaxed Ⓑ. Watch the elbow so your head turns as well, and keep hips facing front with knees slightly bent. Bring arm to front again, then change to other side. Do 10 reps (5 each side), then rest before doing another 2 sets.

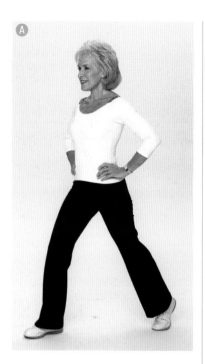

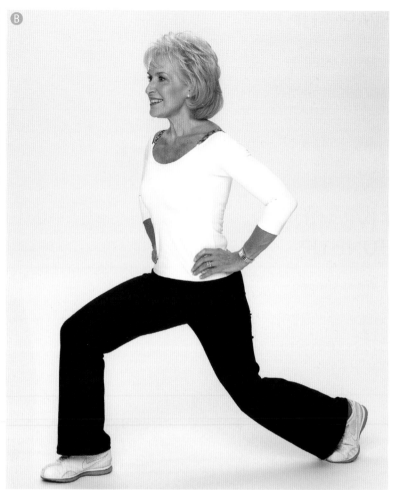

2 Thigh toner ▲ ▶

(2 × 10 reps alternate legs)
Stand tall with hands on hips and tummy in. Now take a large step forward Ⓐ, then dip down, bending both knees, with front knee at a 90-degree angle and directly over ankle Ⓑ. Step back again to bring feet together, then step out with other leg. Do 10 reps (5 each leg), then rest before doing another set.

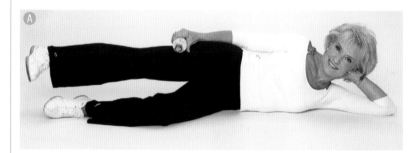

3 Outer thigh shaper ▶

(3 × 16 reps each leg)
Lie on side, bend bottom leg up to 90 degrees and push top leg out straight in line with hip, with foot flexed. Hold a weight or water bottle on the thigh Ⓐ. Pull your tummy in to hold your trunk still, then lift top leg under control Ⓑ, and slowly lower again. Keep lifting and lowering leg for 16 reps, then roll over and repeat with other leg. Rest before doing another 2 sets.

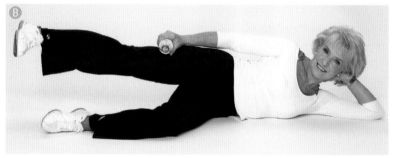

4 Posture improver ▶

(2 × 8 reps)

Lie on front with both arms out to sides at right angles and elbows in line with shoulders. Keeping your head down and relaxed, lift bent arms off floor (if this is too difficult, just lift elbows). Lower again, and repeat. Do 8 reps, then rest before repeating another set.

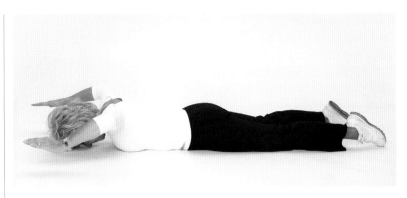

5 Spine strengthener ▶

(3 × 6 reps)

Lie on front with elbows close to waist and palms facing up Ⓐ. Now breathe in and, as you breathe out, lift head and shoulders just off floor, keeping head facing floor Ⓑ. Pause for 2 seconds, then release. Do 6 reps, then rest before doing another 2 sets.

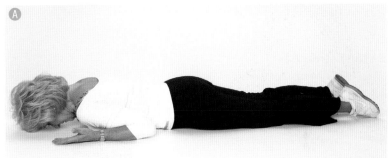

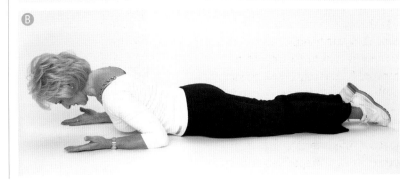

POST-WORKOUT STRETCHES

1 Front thigh stretch ▶

Lie on front, bend one knee and take hold of foot with hand on same side (or hold on to trouser leg or sock). Relax your upper body and gently press your hip into floor to feel a stretch down front of thigh. Hold for 10 seconds, then change legs and repeat.

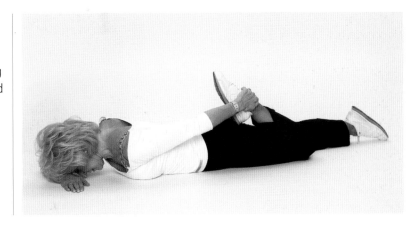

2 Back stretch ▶

Come up onto your hands and knees and, as you pull your tummy in, arch your spine up towards ceiling, letting your head drop down. Hold for 10 seconds, then release.

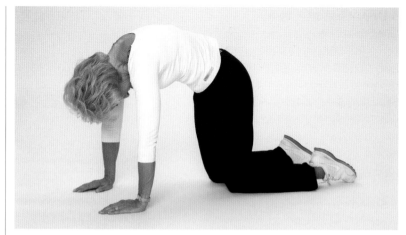

3 Waist stretch ▶

Sit up tall with legs crossed, lift right arm and lean over to left side, keeping both hips on floor and without leaning forward or back. Hold for 10 seconds, then change sides and repeat.

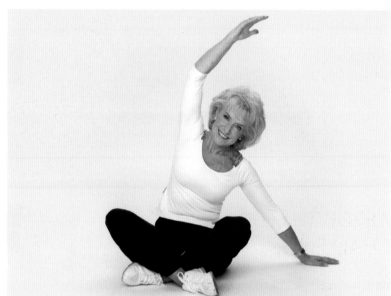

4 Outer thigh and hip ▶ stretch

Sit upright with legs straight out in front and bring left foot over right leg, placing foot flat on floor. Place left hand on floor for support and right hand across left knee. Use pressure of right arm to pull left leg further across body to feel a stretch in outer thigh and hip. Hold for 10 seconds, then change legs and repeat.

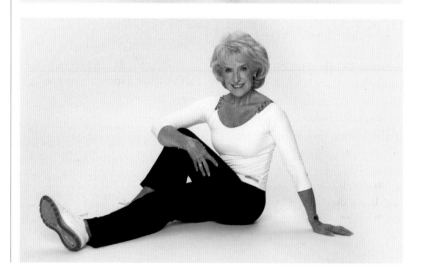

5 Upper back stretch ▶

Sit up tall with legs crossed, bring both arms forward at shoulder height and clasp hands. Drop your head forward to feel a stretch in back of neck, then gently press your upper back away from hands to feel a stretch in upper back. Hold for 10 seconds, then release.

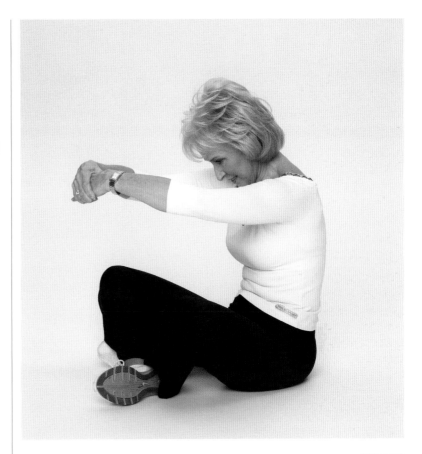

AEROBIC CHALLENGE

Work out for 30–40 minutes at an aerobics class or to one of my aerobic fitness DVDs (my latest Real Results Workout DVD is a great fat burner). Alternatively, go for a 40-minute brisk walk.

Exercise tip
Wearing wrist and ankle weights makes our arm and leg muscles work harder during toning exercises, but we should never use them during aerobic exercise as they can place too much strain on the joints, particularly the shoulders, or cause us to trip.

MOTIVATIONAL THOUGHT FOR THE DAY

Did you know that one pound of body fat is equivalent to half a litre of oil? So when you get weighed tomorrow, really appreciate every single extra pound that you have lost this week.

The great news is that, even after you have finished the 14-Day Fast Track, you will continue to lose weight at a very healthy and encouraging rate of two or three pounds per week while enjoying a more generous calorie allowance in weeks three and four.

Your body should be feeling comfortable with the amount of calories it is receiving – it won't feel it is starving and your metabolic rate should be staying buoyant, particularly in view of the amount of exercise you are doing. Remember, aerobic exercise raises the metabolic rate and it stays elevated for several hours afterwards, while toning exercises encourage stronger, energy-hungry muscles, which also results in a higher metabolic rate, so it's a win/win situation all round.

Day 14

Only one day to go to the end of the 14-Day Fast Track and your second weigh-in. Tomorrow's results will probably not be as significant as last week's because in the first seven days of dieting some of the weight you lose will be fluid. By week two your fluid levels will have evened out, so what you are losing now is real, unadulterated body fat. However, the tape measure will tell you how many inches you have lost – and hence give you an indication of how much body fat has disappeared – and this should give you lots of encouragement.

Today, stay focused and avoid snacking at all costs. Work hard at your aerobic exercise and aim to complete all the reps in today's toning exercises, which work the abdominals, backside, front thighs, chest and upper arms and shoulders.

Try not to go food shopping until after you have weighed and measured yourself tomorrow, so you are not led into temptation. Have a great day.

MENU

Breakfast
■ Fruit Smoothie: blend 150g fresh fruit (peaches, strawberries, raspberries or blueberries) with 100g Total 2% fat Greek Yoghurt and milk from allowance ☑

Mid-morning power snack
■ 1 kid's fun-size mini banana ☑

Lunch
■ 1 × 175g oven-baked sweet potato, topped with 75g baked beans and served with a side salad tossed in low-fat dressing of your choice ☑

Mid-afternoon power snack
■ 1 small apple ☑

Dinner
■ Mixed Grill: 4 turkey rashers and 1 low-fat sausage, grilled, served with 1 dry-fried egg, 1 yellow Portion Pot® (115g) baked beans, unlimited grilled mushrooms plus 1 × 400g can tomatoes boiled well to reduce **P**
OR
■ 3-egg omelette made using milk from allowance and cooked in a non-stick pan. Add 25g grated Rosemary Conley low-fat Mature Cheese and 25g shredded ham or chicken. Serve with a large salad tossed in fat-free dressing **P**

WARM-UP

Twisted canoeing

Stand tall and bring both arms overhead with tummy in. Now drop both arms to one side as you bend your knees and hips, then come up and repeat, dropping your arms to the other side. Keep going for 1 minute.

FIVE-MINUTE TONE-UP

1 Slow tummy curls ▶

(× 6 reps)

Lie on back with knees bent, feet flat on floor and hip width apart, and place both hands behind head. Pull your tummy in and breathe in and, as you breathe out, lift head and shoulders off floor, keeping a distance between chin and chest Ⓐ. Breathe in as you bring left arm forward Ⓑ then the right arm Ⓒ. Breathe out as you put left arm back behind head Ⓓ, followed by right arm, then lower head to floor. Keep your tummy pulled in throughout. Do 6 reps altogether.

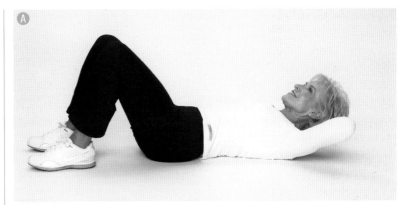

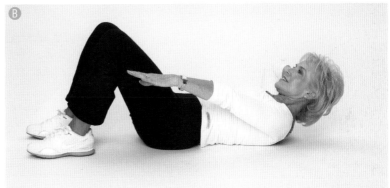

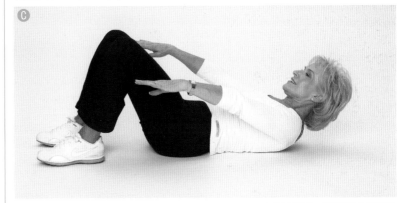

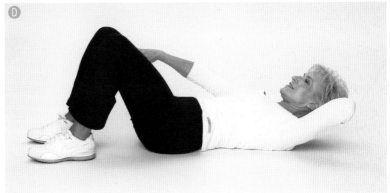

2 One side hip lift ▶

(2 × 6 reps each leg)

Still lying on back, rest one ankle on opposite knee and place arms by sides. Bring heel of other foot a little closer to hips Ⓐ. Now breathe in and, as you breathe out, lift hips off floor without arching your back Ⓑ. Lower again slowly and do 6 reps on same side, then change legs and repeat. Rest, then do another set.

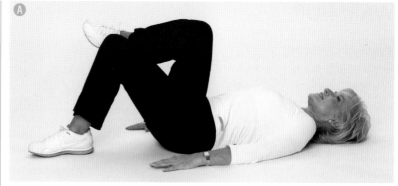

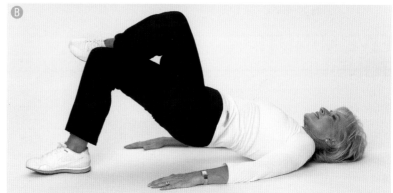

3 Chest and underarm ▶ toner

(2 × 10 reps)

Come up onto hands and knees with wrists in line with shoulders and your knees directly under hips Ⓐ. Pull tummy in to support your back, then breathe in and bend elbows, taking forehead towards floor Ⓑ. Breathe out and come up again without locking elbows at top. Do 10 reps, then rest before doing another set.

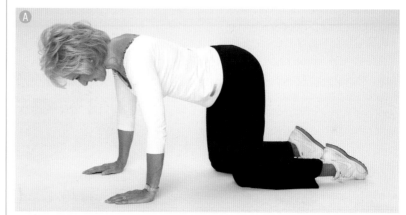

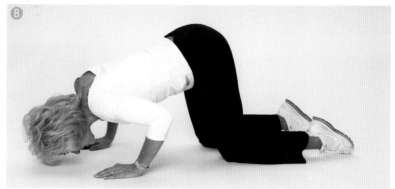

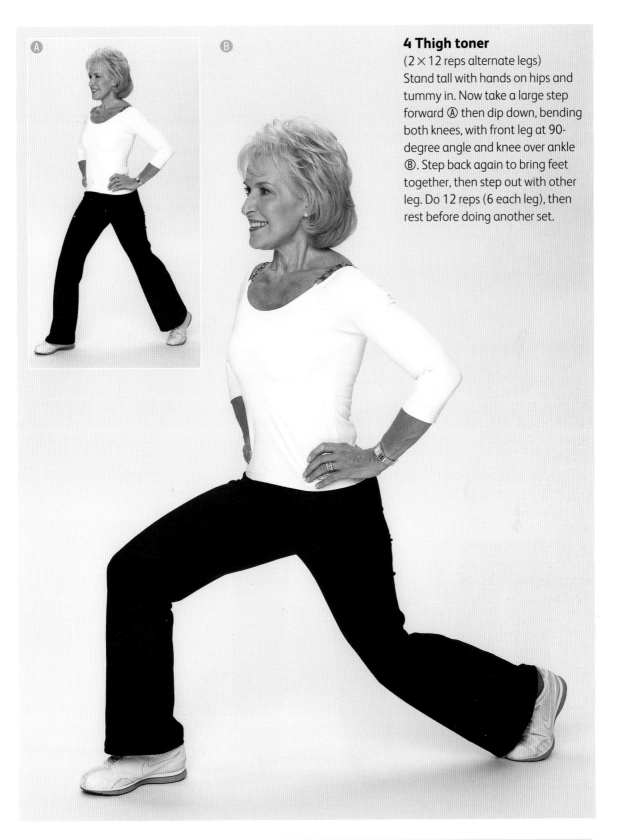

4 Thigh toner

(2 × 12 reps alternate legs)
Stand tall with hands on hips and tummy in. Now take a large step forward Ⓐ then dip down, bending both knees, with front leg at 90-degree angle and knee over ankle Ⓑ. Step back again to bring feet together, then step out with other leg. Do 12 reps (6 each leg), then rest before doing another set.

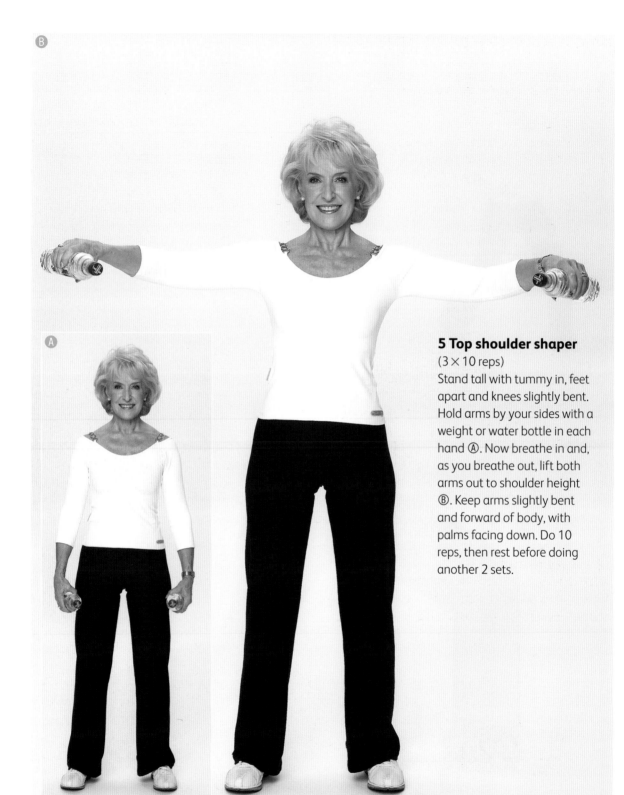

5 Top shoulder shaper
(3 × 10 reps)
Stand tall with tummy in, feet apart and knees slightly bent. Hold arms by your sides with a weight or water bottle in each hand Ⓐ. Now breathe in and, as you breathe out, lift both arms out to shoulder height Ⓑ. Keep arms slightly bent and forward of body, with palms facing down. Do 10 reps, then rest before doing another 2 sets.

POST-WORKOUT STRETCHES

1 Back thigh and bottom stretch

Lie on back with both knees bent and take hold behind one leg, placing one hand at back of thigh and other hand on calf. Keeping both hips firmly on floor, straighten leg as much as possible and hold for 10 seconds. Then try to straighten leg more for a further 10 seconds. Change legs and repeat.

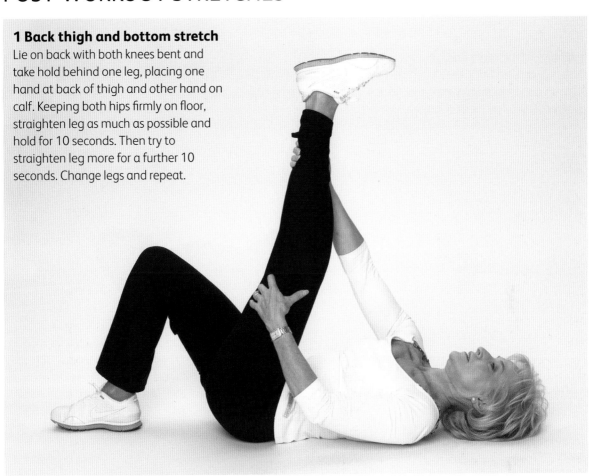

2 Tummy stretch

Lie on back with legs straight and take arms overhead. Stretch arms away from legs to feel a stretch down your tummy. Hold stretch for 10 seconds.

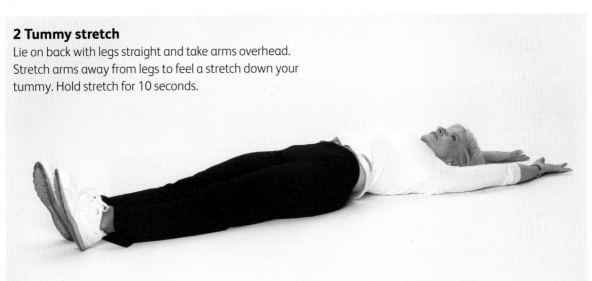

3 Underarm stretch ▶

Sit upright with legs crossed and place right hand behind right shoulder. Press left hand on right underarm to push right hand further down your back. Keep your head up and look straight ahead. Hold for 10 seconds, then change arms and repeat.

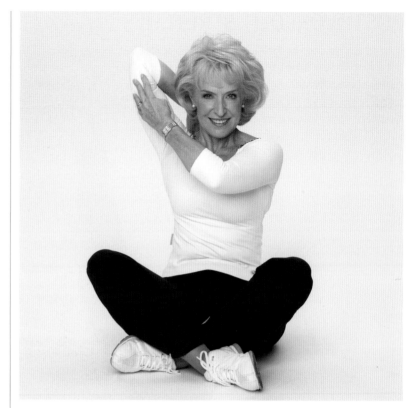

4 Shoulder stretch ▶

Bring right arm across your body at shoulder height. Use other arm to gently press on upper arm to stretch outside of shoulder. Hold for 10 seconds, then change arms and repeat.

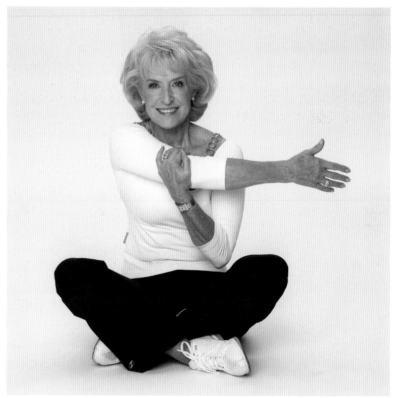

5 Chest stretch ▶

Sit upright and place both hands behind you on floor. Draw shoulders back to feel a stretch across chest, and hold for 10 seconds.

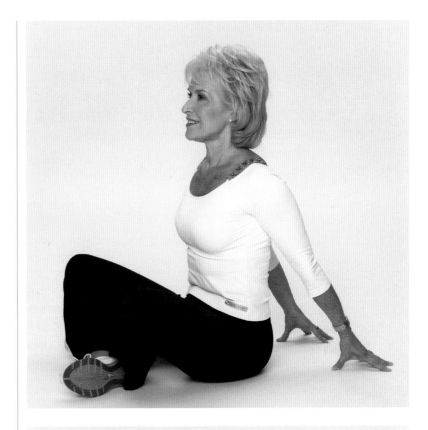

AEROBIC CHALLENGE

Take a 30–40 minute brisk walk or work out to a fitness DVD for 30–40 minutes. Don't forget to stretch afterwards.

Exercise tip

Did you know that we burn twice as many calories standing up than we do sitting down? So try to stand up when you are making phone calls or chatting.

MOTIVATIONAL THOUGHT FOR THE DAY

Today is a very important day. If you have managed to get to the end of this tough fortnight, with its restricted-calorie diet, and you've refrained from drinking alcohol and eating chocolate and completed the exercises every day, you are a star! Well done. You have achieved a significant goal and this will have boosted your self-esteem and confidence. Brilliant!

First thing tomorrow morning, after you have visited the bathroom, weigh and measure yourself carefully, then write down all the details in your notebook. Take a good look at yourself in the mirror and congratulate yourself on your progress. Even if you still have some way to go, you have done very, very well to get this far.

Remember not to sabotage your progress now. Keep focused and stay active for this last day of the 14-Day Fast Track.

Phase 2:
Day 15

I hope you are delighted with the results that the scales and the tape measure or Magic Measure® have given you today. Move the portable clips on your Magic Measure® to today's measurements and add your inch losses to your total-inches-lost chart. Remember to try on your measuring belt too. Find your 'this-is-how-much-weight-I've-lost' carrier bag and add to it the appropriate weight of tins or packets of food equal to this week's weight loss. Be proud of your achievements and don't forget to tell your encourager.

From today you will be following the **14-Day 1400** diet and you are allowed an extra 200 calories each day. So you can have a low-fat pudding or some extra fruit up to the value of 100 calories, *plus* an alcoholic drink or a high-fat treat such as a fun-size Twix as long as it has no more than 100 calories.

The eating plan I've suggested for today includes a pudding and a treat of a glass (125ml) of champagne, because you deserve it. I suggest you buy a small bottle of champagne to avoid wastage – and temptation! – or why not invite some friends round to share a larger bottle and toast your success so far? Of course you can swap the champagne for another treat or drink if you want.

The exercises are getting much more challenging now to help you achieve the maximum benefit in this first month of your new diet and fitness regime. Today we'll be targeting the waist, back, inner and outer thighs and the chest and underarms. Do what you can and if you find any of them too tough, do the easier versions that you are already familiar with and then progress to the harder variations later. I have given you a rest day from your aerobics today.

MENU

Breakfast
- 200g Total 2% fat Greek Yoghurt mixed with 1 tsp runny honey ✓

Mid-morning power snack
- 1 whole papaya, peeled and deseeded ✓

Lunch
- Salad Bowl with Prawns, Chicken or Ham: Place a large selection of shredded salad leaves and fresh herbs such as coriander and basil in a serving dish. Add layers of chopped peppers, onion, celery, mushrooms, cucumber and cherry tomatoes and top with chopped fresh fruits such as pineapple, papaya, mango, kiwi. Add 50g cooked prawns or chicken or shredded ham, then pour some low-fat Marie Rose sauce or other low-fat dressing over the salad and sprinkle with chopped chives **P**
OR
- Any pre-packed sandwich (max. 300 kcal and 5% fat) ✓

Mid-afternoon power snack
- 100g cherries ✓

Dinner
- 150g cod fillet, microwaved or steamed, and 50g cooked prawns, served with ½ × 300g pack (150g) Schwartz for Fish low-fat Chunky Tomato, Olive and Rosemary Sauce, plus unlimited carrots and broccoli or courgettes and 1 yellow Portion Pot® (70g) peas **P**
OR
- Southern Fried Turkey (see recipe, p.213) served hot with unlimited vegetables (excluding potatoes) or salad **P**

Dessert
- 1 × 165g Müllerlight vanilla yogurt sprinkled with dark chocolate

Alcohol or high-fat treat
- 1 yellow Portion Pot® (125ml) champagne or white wine
OR
- 1 × 25g bag Walkers Baked Salt & Vinegar crisps ✓

WARM-UP

March on spot with shoulder rolls

Stand tall and march on the spot for a total of 2 minutes. For every 4 steps, do a full shoulder roll, pulling shoulders forward, up, back and down.

FIVE-MINUTE TONE-UP

1 Chest and underarm ▶ toner

(2 × 6 reps)

Start on hands and knees, with hands under shoulders and your knees under hips, then move knees further back and pull tummy in Ⓐ. Breathe in as you lower upper body towards floor, bending elbows outward and leading with chest Ⓑ. Breathe out as you push up again without locking elbows. Do 6 reps, then rest and build up to another set.

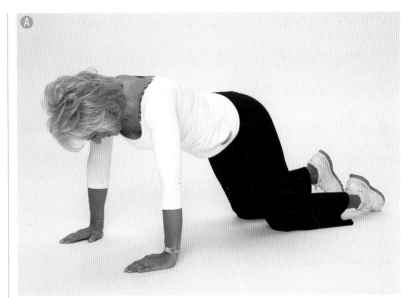

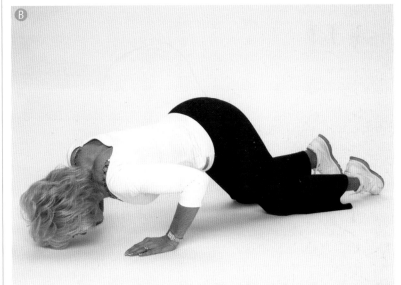

2 Spine strengthener ▶

(2 × 8 reps alternate sides)

Lie on front with arms above head and legs wide. Breathe in and, as you breathe out, lift opposite leg and arm, letting head lift slightly in line with spine. Lower under control, and repeat with other arm and leg. Do 8 reps (4 each side), then rest before doing another set.

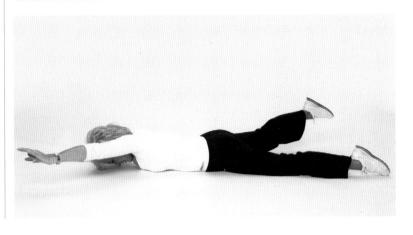

3 Outer thigh shaper with ▶ two-stage lift

(2 × 8 reps each leg)

Lie on side, bend bottom leg up to 90 degrees, push top leg out straight in line with hip, foot flexed, and hold a weight on top thigh. Pull tummy in to hold trunk still, then lift top leg halfway up and pause Ⓐ. Now lift leg higher, keeping hips stacked Ⓑ. Lower again under control, again pausing halfway. Do 8 reps on one leg, then roll over and repeat on other leg. Rest before doing another set.

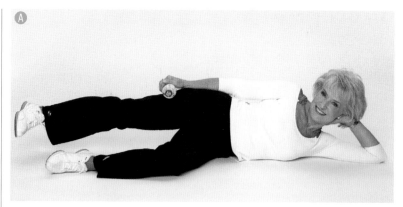

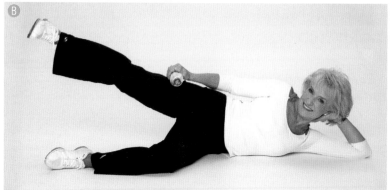

4 Repeated waist twist ▶

(× 10 reps each side)

Lie on back with hands behind head and place left ankle on right knee Ⓐ. Breathe in and, as you breathe out, pull tummy in tight and lift right shoulder in direction of left knee Ⓑ. Lower again and keep repeating to same side for 10 reps, then change sides and repeat.

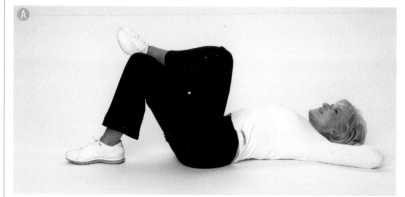

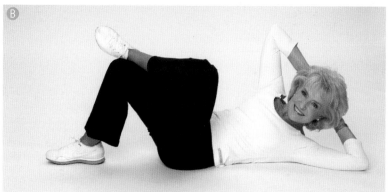

5 Inner thigh toner with ▶ two-stage lift

(2 × 8 reps each leg)

Lie on side propped up on elbow, with top leg bent over bottom leg and knee resting on a rolled towel. Straighten bottom leg and keep it off floor slightly Ⓐ. Pulling tummy in to keep trunk still, lift bottom leg halfway up and pause Ⓑ, then lift to top of range Ⓒ before lowering again with a pause halfway down. Do 8 reps, then rest before doing another set. Change legs and repeat.

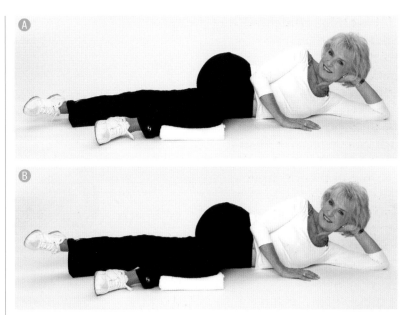

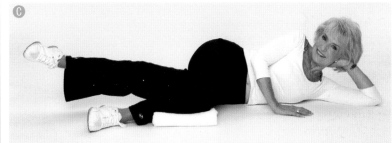

POST-WORKOUT STRETCHES

1 Waist stretch ▶

Sitting up tall with legs crossed, lift right arm and lean over to left side, keeping both hips on floor and without leaning forward or back. Hold for 10 seconds, then change legs and repeat.

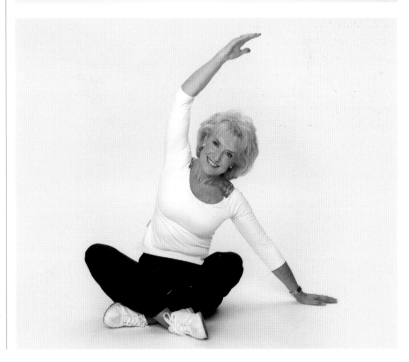

2 Inner thigh stretch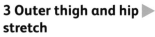

Sit upright with soles of feet together and elbows resting on inside of thighs. Keeping your head up and back straight, lean forward and press elbows onto thighs. Hold for 10 seconds, then breathe in and, as you breathe out, press down further on thighs and hold for another 10 seconds.

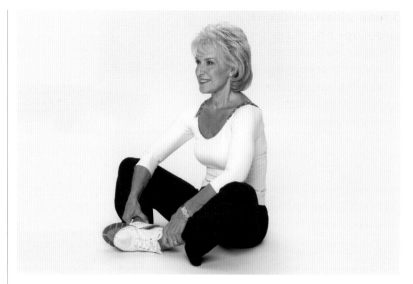

3 Outer thigh and hip stretch

Sit upright with legs straight out in front and bring left foot over right leg, placing foot flat on floor. Place left hand on floor for support and right hand across left knee. Use pressure of right arm to pull left leg further across body to feel a stretch in outer thigh and hip. Hold for 10 seconds, then change legs and repeat.

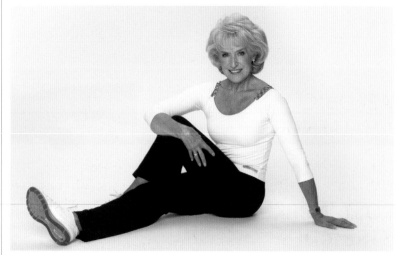

4 Chest stretch

Sit upright and place both hands behind you on floor. Draw shoulders back to feel a stretch across chest, and hold for 10 seconds.

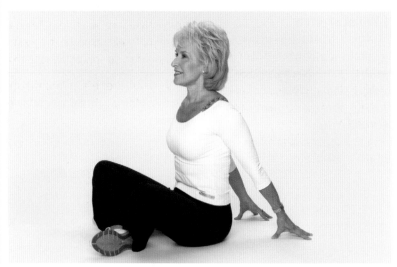

5 Back stretch ▶

Come up onto hands and knees and, as you pull tummy in, arch your spine up towards the ceiling, letting your head drop down. Hold for 10 seconds, then release.

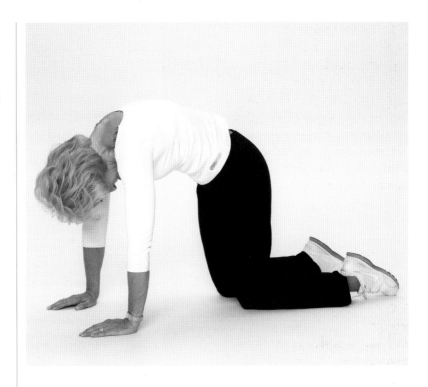

AEROBIC CHALLENGE

Go for a brisk 30-minute walk or work out to a fitness DVD for 30 minutes. Also, walk up and down stairs 4 times consecutively, twice during the day.

Exercise tip

By parking your car further away at the supermarket you are more likely to find a space and avoid getting your car scratched or dented. You will have walked extra steps towards your fitness and slimness too!

MOTIVATIONAL THOUGHT FOR THE DAY

'Nothing succeeds like success', so the proverb goes, and now that your weight and inch loss progress has taken a huge leap forward you should settle comfortably into the second phase of this weight loss programme.

While the next two weeks will be slightly easier because you have an extra couple of hundred calories each day to play with, in order to maximise your weight and inch loss, I want you to pep up your activity levels. In any case, you will be feeling fitter by now, as well as lighter, so you should be able to do more without feeling exhausted.

Put every bit of effort into this next 14 days and in two weeks' time you will have achieved a massive turnaround in your health and fitness. Enjoy it.

Day 16

I hope you enjoyed your alcoholic drink or high-fat treat yesterday and that it had a positive effect of making you feel good rather than frustrated that you couldn't have more! Some people find it easier to abstain completely rather than dice with temptation – once they have the taste of the alcohol or chocolate they find it difficult to stop – while others find that having a little of what they fancy is enough to keep them satisfied. I fall into the second category. I am quite happy to have a few chips from my husband Mike's plate, or just a spoonful of someone else's delicious dessert (Mike doesn't do desserts!). Fortunately I have an understanding husband and accommodating friends! So, recognise which sort of personality you are and plan accordingly. Avoid temptation and play to your strengths.

Try to do today's aerobic challenge with extra vigour so you burn even more calories and fat. Today's toning workout uses a dining chair and concentrates on the abdominals and hips and thighs. Your muscles are working much harder now, which will really help to tone your body. Remember to drink plenty of water or low-cal drinks to stay hydrated.

MENU

Breakfast
- 2 Quorn sausages, grilled, served with 1 × 400g can tomatoes boiled until reduced, plus 50g grilled mushrooms ✓ P

Mid-morning power snack
- 1 × 90g pack Tesco Fresh Apple and Grape Snack Pack ✓

Lunch
- Mixed Bean Salad: Mix together 100g drained, canned chickpeas, 100g red kidney beans and 25g sweetcorn kernels. Add 2 sliced spring onions, 3 halved cherry tomatoes, unlimited chopped celery, peppers and cucumber, and mix well. Stir in some chopped fresh coriander and basil and toss in balsamic vinegar or fat-free dressing of your choice and add freshly ground black pepper to taste ✓
OR
- 1 pack Rosemary Conley Solo Slim Soup: choose from Tomato, Pea and Ham, Three Bean and Chorizo, Mushroom or Minestrone (order from www.rosemaryconley.com). Plus 1 slice wholegrain bread and 1 piece fresh fruit ✓

Mid-afternoon power snack
- 1 rice cake spread with 20g Philadelphia Extra Light soft cheese and sliced cucumber ✓

Dinner
- ½ pack any branded fresh filled pasta (max. 5 % fat) served with ½ pot readymade low-fat fresh tomato-based sauce (max. 400 kcal total for whole meal) ✓
OR
- Lamb Medallions with Blackcurrant Sauce (see recipe, p.214) served with 100g boiled new potatoes (with skins) and unlimited vegetables

Dessert
- 1 Marks & Spencer meringue basket filled with 1 tsp 0 % fat Greek yogurt and topped with 3 sliced strawberries ✓

Alcohol or high-fat treat
- 50ml measure of any spirit plus a Slimline mixer
OR
- 1 fun-size Twix

WARM-UP

Ski swings
Stand tall and lift both arms overhead, pulling your tummy in. Now swing arms down and past thighs as you bend knees and hips. Keep your back straight and keep looking forward. Come up again and repeat ski swings for 1 minute.

FIVE-MINUTE TONE-UP

1 Two-stage chair squat
(2 × 8 reps)
Stand in front of a sturdy chair with feet hip width apart and hands on hips Ⓐ. Pull tummy in tight, then bend hips back as if to sit down, but stop halfway to pause Ⓑ. Hold for just a second, then lower hips further to just off chair seat Ⓒ. Come up again, stopping halfway to pause. Do 8 reps, then rest before doing another set.

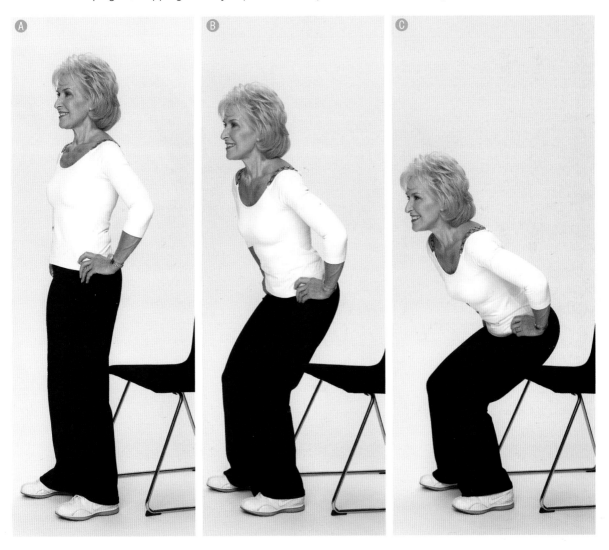

2 Bottom lift ▶

(2 × 8 reps)

Lie on back with arms by sides, legs well bent and lower legs resting on chair seat Ⓐ. Pulling your tummy in, breathe in and, as you breathe out, lift hips off floor, holding tummy in and keeping neck and shoulders relaxed Ⓑ. Do 8 reps, then rest before doing another set.

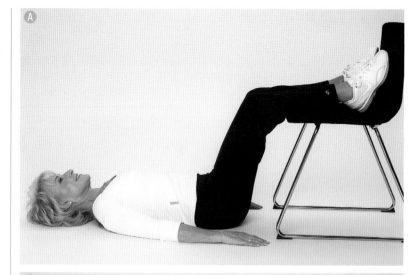

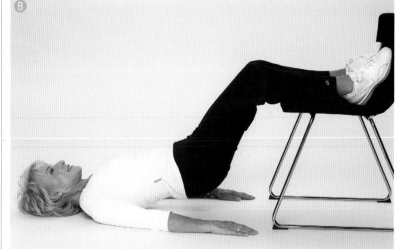

3 Waist trimmer ▶

(2 × 10 reps alternate sides)

Still lying on back with lower legs supported on chair seat, place both hands behind head. Pulling tummy in very tight, breathe in and, as you breathe out, lift left shoulder towards right thigh, keeping elbows wide. Lower again under control with tummy still pulled in, then lift to other side. Do 10 reps (5 each side), then rest before doing another set.

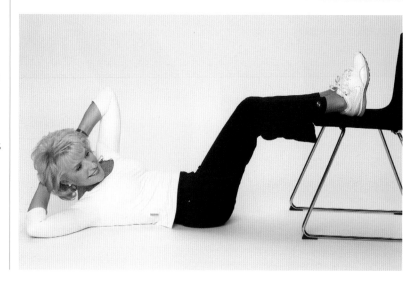

4 Tummy curl ▶

(2 × 12 reps)

Lying on back with lower legs supported on chair seat and hands behind head, pull tummy in very tight and breathe in. As you breathe out, lift head and shoulders off floor and look forward. Lower again under control with tummy still pulled in. Do 12 reps, then rest before doing another set.

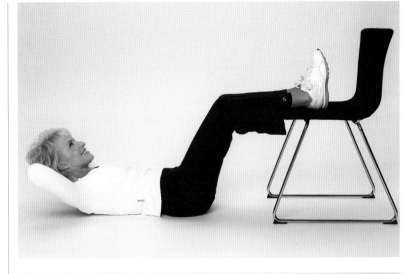

5 Inner thigh toner ▶

(2 × 12 reps each leg)

Lie on side with top leg resting on chair seat and bottom leg on floor Ⓐ. Pull tummy in to hold trunk still, then lift bottom foot under chair seat Ⓑ. Lower again under control. Do 12 reps, then rest before doing another set. Roll over and repeat on other leg.

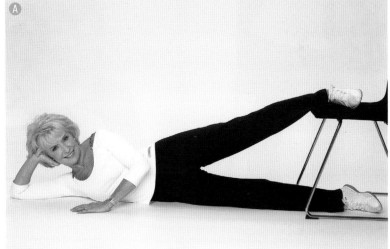

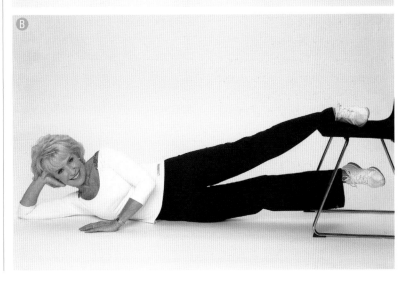

POST-WORKOUT STRETCHES

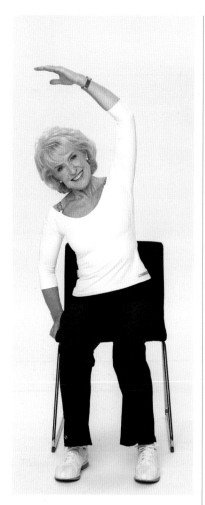

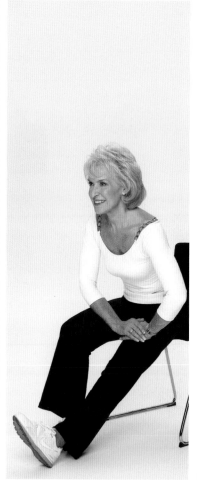

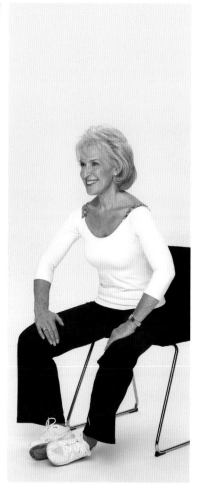

1 Waist stretch ▲

Sit on front third of chair seat and lift left arm, keeping right hand on chair seat for support. Now, keeping both hips firmly on chair seat, bend to right without leaning forward or back and feel a stretch down left side. Hold for 10 seconds, then change sides and repeat.

2 Back thigh stretch ▲

Sit on front third of chair seat and straighten left leg with both hands resting on thigh. Now, keeping your back straight and looking forward, lean from hips to feel a stretch in back of thigh. Hold for 10 seconds, then change legs and repeat.

3 Inner thigh stretch ▲

Still sitting on chair, bend knees and bring feet together, then press hands on inside of thighs to push knees outwards but keeping feet in contact with each other. Hold stretch for 10 seconds, then release.

4 Front thigh stretch

Stand and hold on to back of chair with right hand. Take hold of left ankle with left hand (or hold trouser leg or sock) and bring knees in line with each other. Now press hip of raised leg forward to feel a stretch down front of thigh and hold for 10 seconds. Change sides and repeat on other leg.

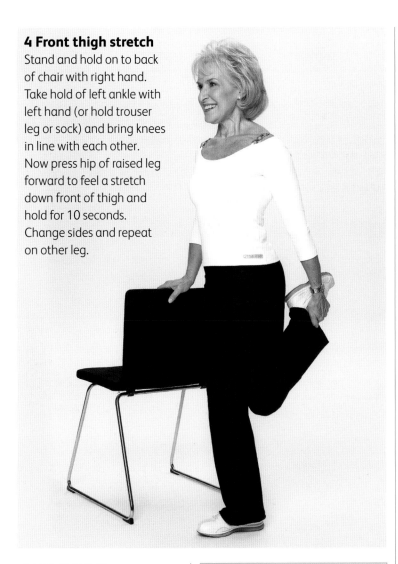

AEROBIC CHALLENGE

Power walk for 30 minutes, swinging your bent arms as you walk. Increase the pace now that you are slimmer and fitter!

Exercise tip

What activities or sport did you enjoy doing at school? What were you good at? Can you find someone to participate in a similar activity with you now? The key to fitness success is finding a form of exercise that you enjoy, because you are likely to do it more often. Give it some thought today and search out that tennis or badminton racquet, buy a football, a skipping rope or a hula hoop!

MOTIVATIONAL THOUGHT FOR THE DAY

Following a low-fat, low-Gi, calorie-controlled eating plan means you won't be depositing unnecessary fat around your body. Combining this way of eating with regular exercise that tones you up as you slim down is not that difficult. It's a question of mindset and once you've followed this lifestyle for 28 days you will have acquired a new habit – one that will dramatically enhance your future health. If eating healthily and taking regular exercise becomes your new lifestyle, you will be making a priceless investment in your future. And you should never have to go on a diet later in life because you will be maintaining a healthy pattern of eating and activity every day as a matter of course.

The great thing about our Diet and Fitness Clubs is that we offer a workout at every class, so members still have a reason for coming even after they have reached their goal weight. I still teach my own classes in Leicester and about 15 of my members have been coming along on a Monday evening for more than 20 years! For them it's a fun night out that helps them to stay focused on eating sensibly and staying fit. The result is they enjoy good health and fit bodies.

Day 17

Do you have a pedometer? If you do, wear it every day to check how active you are. Aim to achieve 10,000 steps a day, or at least 2000 more steps than your usual number, as this will help you to lose your excess weight and also to maintain it once you have achieved a healthy weight. Children should aim to do even more steps a day for good health. If you don't own a pedometer, check out www.rosemaryconley.com for an easy-to-use version that is cheap and effective. I find wearing a pedometer extremely motivating as it encourages me to move about more.

Are you still doing well on the diet? Should you get really peckish, rather than eating something you'll regret later, nibble on some chopped carrots and celery sprinkled with celery salt and have a low-calorie drink. Sometimes feelings of hunger can be confused with thirst.

Today's toning exercises work the abdominals, back muscles, thighs, shoulders, chest and underarms. If you can manage the recommended number of sets and reps, you will be doing very well and the benefits to your body will be huge.

MENU

Breakfast
- 1 small banana, sliced, mixed with 115g sliced strawberries and 1 × 100g pot low-fat yogurt, any flavour (max. 100 kcal and 5% fat) ✔

Mid-morning power snack
- 5 mini low-fat bread sticks plus 1 tsp 0% fat Greek yogurt mixed with chopped chives ✔

Lunch
- Spread 2 slices wholegrain bread with horseradish sauce or Hellmann's Extra Light Mayonnaise and make into a jumbo sandwich with 30g wafer thin beef, chicken or ham, plus salad vegetables
OR
- Bombay Rice (see recipe, p.220) served with salad ✔

Mid-afternoon power snack
- 1 red Portion Pot® (115g) raspberries plus 50g strawberries ✔

Dinner
- Chilli Prawn or Quorn Stir-Fry with Asparagus: Dry-fry ½ chopped red onion and ½ crushed garlic clove in a non-stick pan until soft. Add 50g sliced asparagus and either 100g uncooked, shelled prawns or Quorn pieces and continue cooking for 2–3 minutes. Pour in 1 × 75g pack chilli stir-fry sauce and stir well to coat the prawns and vegetables. Bring to the boil, then turn off the heat. Serve with salad and garnish with fresh chives ✔ **P**
OR
- 1 × 300g pack Rosemary Conley Solo Slim Beef Meatballs and Potato (order from www.rosemaryconley.com) served with unlimited vegetables (excluding potatoes)

Dessert
- 1 Marks & Spencer meringue nest filled with 1 tbsp 0% fat Greek yogurt and topped with 1 tbsp fresh raspberries or blueberries ✔

Alcohol or high-fat treat
- 75ml measure of sweet sherry
OR
- 1 × 19g bag Cheese & Onion Flavour Pom-Bear Teddy-shaped Potato Snacks ✔

WARM-UP

Stair step-ups

Using a single step (such as the bottom step of your stairs), step up and down for 2 minutes. Lead with the right leg for 1 minute, then pause and change to lead with the left leg. Make sure the whole foot makes contact on each step.

FIVE-MINUTE TONE-UP

1 Top shoulder shaper ▼

(3 × 10 reps)

Stand tall with tummy in, feet apart and knees slightly bent. Hold arms by your sides with a weight or water bottle in each hand Ⓐ. Now breathe in and, as you breathe out, lift both arms out to shoulder height Ⓑ. Keep arms slightly bent and forward of body, with palms facing down. Do 10 reps, then rest before doing another 2 sets.

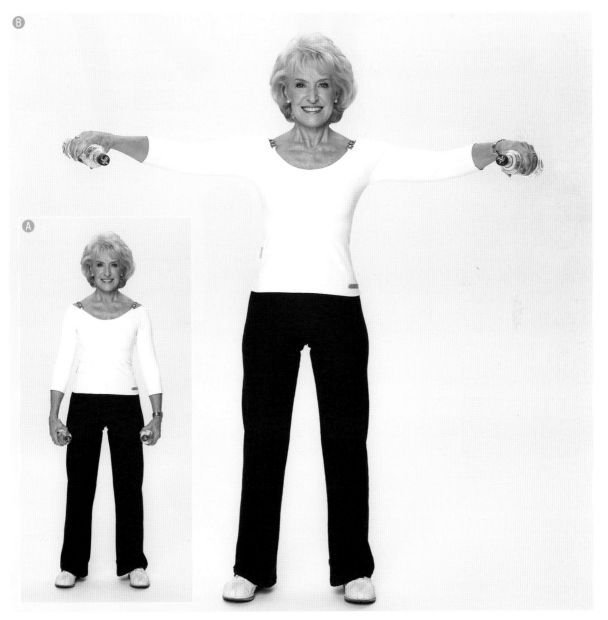

2 Squats with outer leg lift ▶

(2 × 12 reps alternate legs)
Stand tall with feet parallel and hip width apart, hands on hips and tummy in. Now, keeping your back straight, bend knees and hips Ⓐ, then as you come up again, lift one leg out to side, pulling thigh outwards Ⓑ. Bend again, then lift other leg out to side, keeping your trunk upright. Keep changing sides for 12 reps (6 each side), then rest before doing another set. This is great for developing balance, but if you struggle, then hold on to the back of a chair.

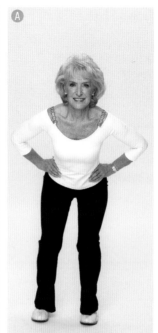
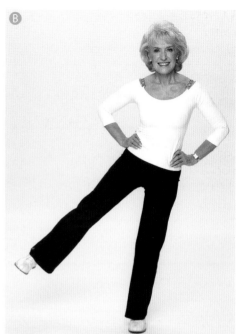

3 Reverse tummy curl ▶

(2 × 8 reps)
Lie on back with legs raised, ankles crossed, palms face up on floor and tummy pulled in tight Ⓐ. Breathe in and, as you breathe out, lift hips off floor, bringing knees closer to your chest Ⓑ. Keep your neck and shoulders relaxed and tummy held in. Do 8 reps slowly, then rest before doing another set.

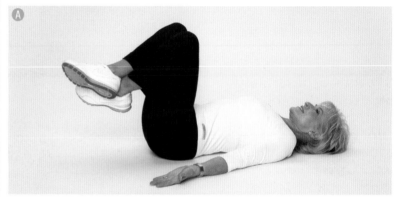

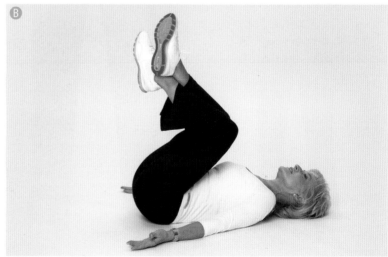

4 Chest and underarm ▶ toner

(2 × 8 reps)

Start on hands and knees, with hands under shoulders and your knees under your hips, then move knees further back and pull tummy in Ⓐ. Breathe in as you lower upper body towards floor, bending elbows outward and leading with chest Ⓑ. Breathe out as you push up again without locking elbows. Do 8 reps, then rest and build up to another set.

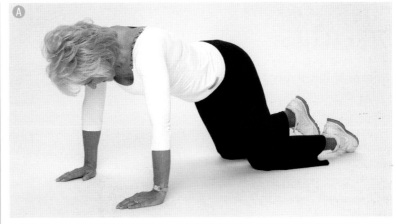

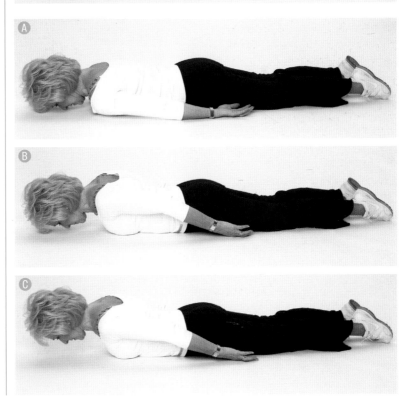

5 Posture improver and ▶ back strengthener

(2 × 6 reps)

Lie on front with arms by sides Ⓐ. Breathe in and, as you breathe out, pull shoulders up away from floor Ⓑ, then lift the head off floor but keep looking down, with head in line with spine Ⓒ. Hold for 2 seconds, then lower slowly. Do 6 reps, then rest before doing another set.

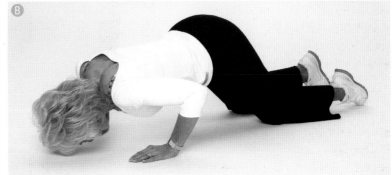

POST-WORKOUT STRETCHES

1 Front thigh stretch ▶

Lie on front, bend one knee and take hold of foot with hand on same side (or hold on to trouser leg or sock). Relax your upper body and gently press hip into floor to feel a stretch down front of thigh. Hold for 10 seconds, then change legs and repeat.

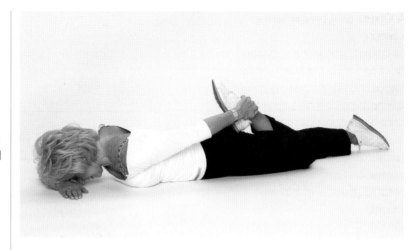

2 Tummy stretch ▶

Lie on front with arms at sides and elbows bent. Now prop up on your elbows, keeping hips in contact with floor, and lift your chin forward slightly to feel a stretch in your tummy. Hold for 10 seconds, then release.

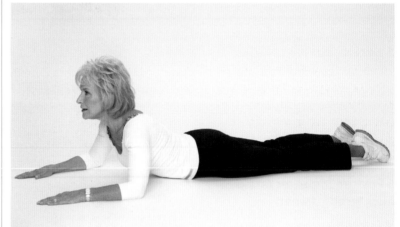

3 Shoulder stretch ▶

Sit upright with legs crossed and bring one arm across trunk at shoulder height. Use other arm to gently press on upper arm to stretch outside of shoulder. Hold for 10 seconds, then change arms and repeat.

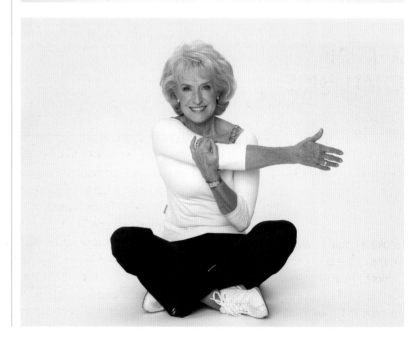

4 Outer thigh and hip ▶ stretch

Sit upright with legs straight out in front and bring left foot over right leg, placing foot flat on floor. Place left hand on floor for support and right hand across left knee. Use pressure of right arm to pull left leg further across body to feel a stretch in outer thigh and hip. Hold for 10 seconds, then change legs and repeat.

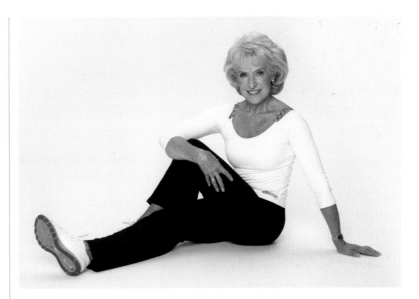

5 Back stretch ▶

Come up onto your hands and knees and, as you pull your tummy in, arch your spine up towards the ceiling, letting your head drop down. Hold for 10 seconds, then release.

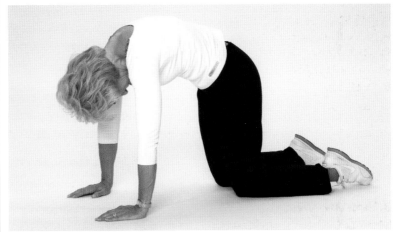

AEROBIC CHALLENGE

If you have a skipping rope, try skipping for as long as you can. March on the spot to give you a chance to get your breath back, then skip some more!

Exercise tip

Make it a rule never to leave items at the bottom of your stairs to take up later. Each trip upstairs will help you to burn extra calories.

MOTIVATIONAL THOUGHT FOR THE DAY

By the time you reach Day 28 you will have developed the habit of eating low-fat, low-Gi foods and being more active in your everyday life. You will automatically choose the stairs in preference to the lift, and leaving the car behind occasionally and walking for those short errands will be second nature. That is what is so brilliant about this 28-day programme. It isn't just a get-slim-quick package, but a lifestyle change programme that can last a lifetime. After you have finished the initial 28 days, if you go back to eating the way you used to, you will regain the weight you have lost. So I really hope this easy way of eating and increased everyday activity becomes a way of life for you so you stay slim and fit for good.

Day 18

One of the benefits of this diet is that every breakfast is interchangeable with every other breakfast in the book. Same with the lunches and also the dinners. There is no need for you to eat anything you don't like or that doesn't fit in with your family's needs. However, it is worth trying new vegetables and other foods that you may not have eaten before. You might be in for some tasty surprises.

Today's toning exercises will trim your waist, strengthen your back and tone your backside, inner thighs and shoulders. Don't rush the exercises and try to 'feel' the muscles working as you perform each move.

MENU

Breakfast
- 1 blue Portion Pot® (35g) uncooked porridge oats, cooked in water with 10 sultanas and served with milk from allowance ☑

Mid-morning power snack
- 1 Asda Good For You Chicken Noodle Cup Soup

Lunch
- Stir-Fry Chicken with Ginger: Chop 100g chicken breast (no skin) into bite-sized pieces and dry-fry in a non-stick pan with ½ crushed garlic clove. When the chicken has changed colour and is almost cooked through, add 1 chopped red or green pepper, 1 chopped celery stick, ½ chopped red onion, 25g mushrooms and 50g mangetout and dry-fry quickly but do not overcook. Just before serving add 1 tsp grated fresh ginger, soy sauce to taste and fresh coriander and heat through **P**
OR
- 1 × 175g oven-baked sweet potato topped with 75g baked beans and served with a side salad tossed in low-fat dressing of your choice ☑

Mid-afternoon power snack
- 75g fresh mango ☑

Dinner
- 1 × 115g salmon steak (raw weight), steamed or microwaved, served with 80g boiled new potatoes (with skins), 1 yellow Portion Pot® (70g) peas, plus 100g broccoli or asparagus and 1 tbsp Hellmann's Extra Light Mayonnaise
OR
- Any low-fat vegetarian ready meal (max. 400 kcal and 5% fat, including any accompaniments) ☑

Dessert
- 1 × 120g pot Danone Shape Fat Free Feel Fuller For Longer yogurt, any flavour ☑

Alcohol or high-fat treat
- 100ml measure of Martini Extra Dry plus Slimline mixer
OR
- 2 Weight Watchers Double Choc Chip Cookies ☑

WARM-UP

March on spot with tummy pull-ins

Stand tall and march on the spot, letting the arms swing naturally. Every 10 steps, really pull your tummy in tight and then relax it for 10 steps.

FIVE-MINUTE TONE-UP

1 Front shoulder shaper ▶

(2 × 10 reps)
Stand tall with back straight and hold a weight or water bottle in each hand, with backs of hands facing forward Ⓐ. Now breathe in and, as you breathe out, lift arms in front to shoulder height, keeping your shoulders down, head up and elbows slightly bent Ⓑ. Lower again slowly, and repeat. Do 10 reps, then rest before doing another set.

2 Inner thigh toner ▶ with two-stage lift

(2 × 12 reps each leg)
Lie on side propped up on elbow, with top leg bent over bottom leg and knee resting on a rolled towel. Straighten bottom leg and keep it off floor slightly Ⓐ. Pulling tummy in to keep trunk still, lift bottom leg halfway up and pause Ⓑ, then lift to top of range Ⓒ before lowering again with a pause halfway down. Do 12 reps, then rest before doing another set. Change legs and repeat.

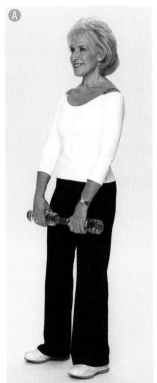
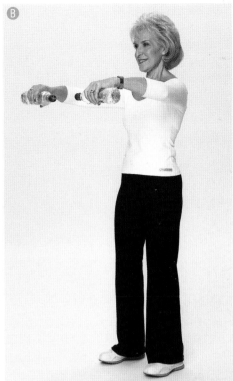
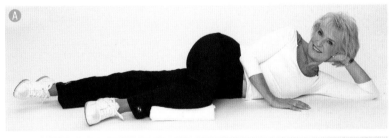
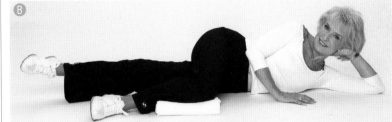
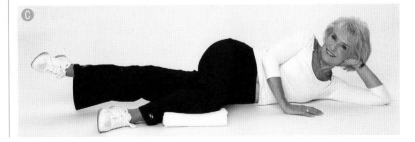

3 Bottom shaper ▶

(2 × 8 reps each leg)

Come up on to forearms and knees and extend one leg behind on floor Ⓐ. Pull tummy in and lift leg to hip height, leading with heel Ⓑ. Lower leg again and continue lifting and lowering, keeping hips facing floor and tummy in tight. Do 8 reps on one leg, then change legs and repeat. Sit back and rest before doing another set.

4 Repeated waist twist ▼

(× 12 reps each side)

Lie on back with hands behind head and place left ankle on right knee. Breathe in and, as you breathe out, pull tummy in tight and lift right shoulder in direction of left knee. Lower again and keep repeating to same side for 12 reps, then change sides and repeat.

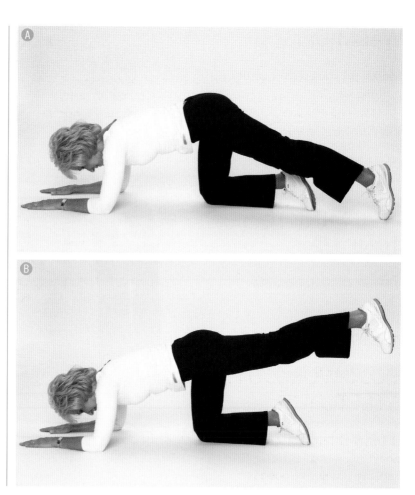

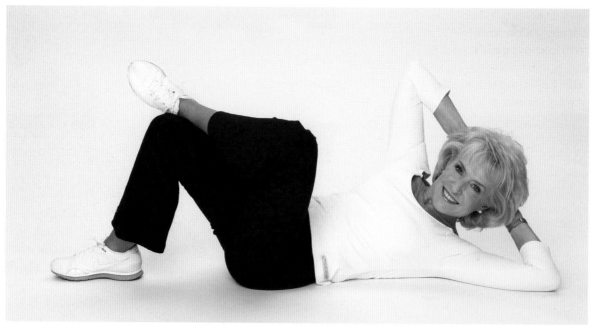

5 Spine strengthener
(3 × 8 reps alternate sides)

Lie on front with arms above head and legs wide. Breathe in and, as you breathe out, lift opposite leg and arm, letting head lift slightly in line with spine. Lower under control, and repeat with other arm and leg. Do 8 reps, then rest before doing another 2 sets.

POST-WORKOUT STRETCHES

1 Inner thigh stretch ▶
Sit upright with soles of feet together and elbows resting on inside of thighs. Keeping your head up and back straight, lean forward and press elbows onto thighs. Hold for 10 seconds, then breathe in and, as you breathe out, press down further on thighs and hold for another 10 seconds.

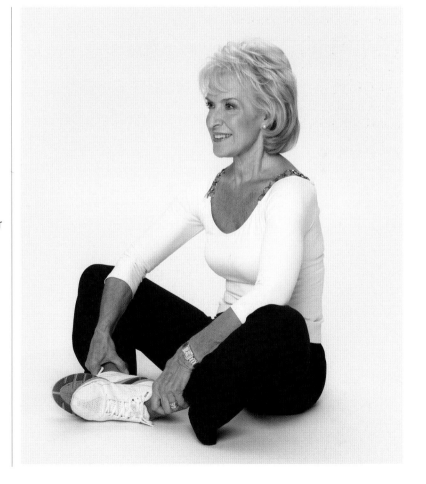

2 Back thigh stretch ▶

Sit upright with one leg straight out in front and the other bent. Place hands on floor at either side of straight leg and lean forward from hips to feel a stretch in back of thigh. Hold for 10 seconds, then try to lean a little further forward for another 10 seconds. Change legs and repeat.

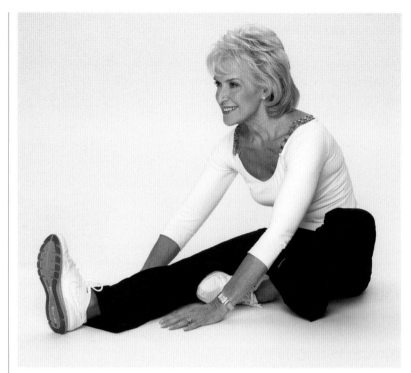

3 Waist stretch ▶

Still sitting up tall with legs crossed, lift right arm and lean over to left side, keeping both hips on floor and without leaning forward or back. Hold for 10 seconds, then change sides and repeat.

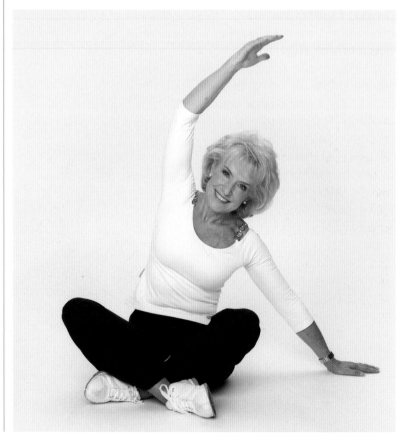

4 Chest stretch ▶

Sit upright and place both hands behind you on floor. Draw shoulders back to feel a stretch across chest, and hold for 10 seconds.

AEROBIC CHALLENGE

Walk up and down stairs 5 times consecutively, then repeat later in the day. In addition, go for a 15-minute brisk walk or work out at a class or to a fitness DVD.

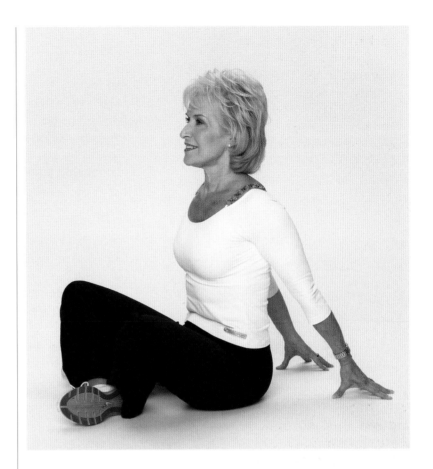

Exercise tip

Did you know that working as a chambermaid is one of the most active jobs you can do? It burns more calories than most other occupations because chambermaids are on their feet most of the day. So, next time you make the beds and do the housework, remember that you are burning calories and, instead of seeing it as a chore, think of it as a workout and do it with extra zeal.

MOTIVATIONAL THOUGHT FOR THE DAY

After today there are only ten days to go before you complete the 28-day programme. What a fantastic achievement that will be and think of how much slimmer you will look and feel compared to when you started the programme. It's difficult to predict the exact rate at which we will lose weight. Sometimes the scales tell us we haven't lost much yet the tape measure shows that we are definitely losing inches. That's why it's worth taking the time to measure yourself once a week so you don't lose heart. All you can do is give it your best effort – so stick to the diet, do the exercises and activities as described and continue to be as active as you can every day. The results will be phenomenal and you will be so pleased you made the effort.

Day 19

Ten days to go and everything to look forward to. Your body is getting used to being fed a healthy diet of smaller quantities of food than previously as well as benefiting from increased levels of activity, and you are reaping the rewards. It's as if your body is giving a huge sigh of relief and thinking 'At last I'm being fed what I need to be healthy!'

It can be quite frightening to realise how much we have abused our bodies over the years and how, despite the bad treatment, they have somehow managed to survive and support us. But only now will you be enjoying the full extent of the benefits of eating a much healthier diet and using your muscles more.

Muscles respond wonderfully to being used and challenged, and exercise is our passport to a longer, more independent, life. There is no downside, providing you are wise about the amount of exercise you do and you listen to your body so you know when you've done enough. Try your best to complete today's toning exercises, which focus on the abdominals, outer thighs and front thighs, chest, underarms and shoulders.

Start enjoying that looser waistband and the extra energy you will be experiencing. Have a good day.

MENU

Breakfast
■ 1 yellow Portion Pot® (14 Minis) Weetabix Fruit 'n' Nut Minis, plus 1 medium-sized banana, sliced, served with milk from allowance ☑

Mid-morning power snack
■ 12 seedless grapes ☑

Lunch
■ 1 medium slice wholegrain bread, toasted, topped with 1 × 125g can sardines or mackerel fillets, plus a small salad
OR
■ 1 can any lentil or bean soup (max. 350 kcal and 5% fat), plus 1 piece fresh fruit (excluding bananas) ☑

Mid-afternoon power snack
■ 10 sweet silverskin pickled onions plus 10 cherry tomatoes ☑

Dinner
■ Chicken or Quorn in Mushroom Sauce: Dry-fry 100g chopped chicken breast (no skin) or Quorn alternative with ½ chopped onion and 6 button mushrooms. When the chicken is almost cooked, add 100g (⅓ can) Batchelors Low Fat Condensed Mushroom Soup, plus milk from allowance if needed to make a creamy sauce. Simmer until the chicken is completely cooked. Serve with 1 yellow Portion Pot® (100g) mashed sweet potato, plus other vegetables of your choice ☑
OR
■ 1 × 300g pack Rosemary Conley Solo Slim Lamb Hotpot (order from www.rosemaryconley.com). Plus 1 low-fat yogurt (max. 150 kcal and 5% fat)

Dessert
■ 1 × 55g pot Asda Great Fruity Stuff fromage frais, any flavour ☑

Alcohol or high-fat treat
■ 300ml (½ pint) dry cider
OR
■ 1 × 23g bag Walkers French Fries Ready Salted crisps ☑

WARM-UP

Knee lifts with pull-downs

Stand upright with hands above head and tummy pulled in. Lift alternate knees and as you lift each knee, pull your arms down to either side of the knees. Keep your tummy in and your back straight and continue for 1 minute.

FIVE-MINUTE TONE-UP

1 Slow tummy curl ▶

(×8 reps)

Lie on your back with knees bent, feet flat on floor and hip width apart and hands behind head. Pull tummy in and breathe in and, as you breathe out, lift head and shoulders off floor, keeping a distance between chin and chest Ⓐ. Breathe in as you bring left arm forward Ⓑ then the right arm Ⓒ. Breathe out as you put left arm back behind head Ⓓ, followed by right arm, then lower head to floor. Keep your tummy pulled in throughout. Do 8 reps altogether.

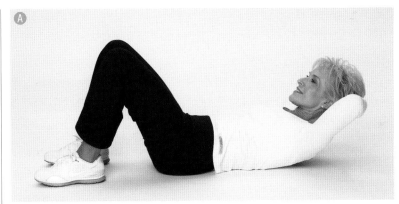

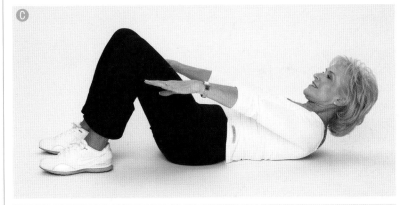

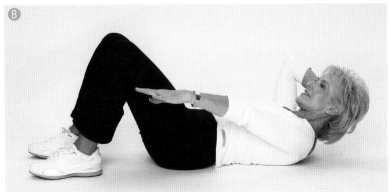

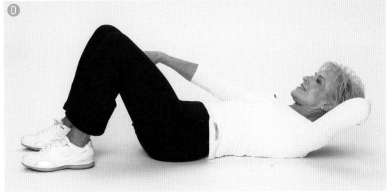

2 Outer thigh shaper ▶ with two-stage lift

(2 × 12 reps each leg)

Lie on side, bend bottom leg up to 90 degrees and push top leg out straight in line with hip, foot flexed, and hold a weight on top thigh. Pull tummy in to hold trunk still, then lift top leg halfway up and pause Ⓐ. Now lift leg higher to top of range, keeping hips stacked Ⓑ. Lower under control, stopping again halfway to pause. Do 12 reps on one leg, then roll over and repeat on other leg. Rest before doing another set.

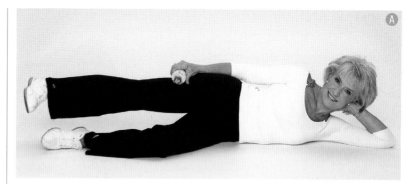

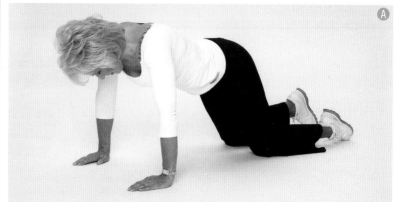

3 Chest and underarm ▶ toner

(2 × 8 reps)

Start on hands and knees, with hands under shoulders and your knees under hips, then move knees further back and pull tummy in Ⓐ. Breathe in as you lower upper body towards floor, bending elbows outward and leading with chest Ⓑ. Breathe out as you push up again without locking elbows. Do 8 reps, then rest and build up to another set.

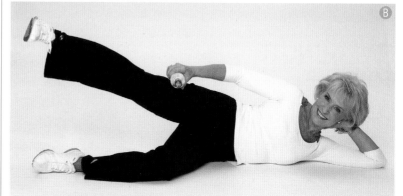

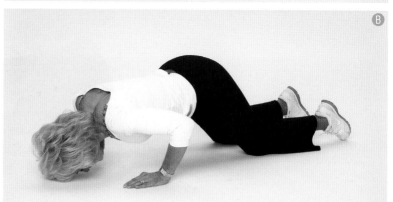

4 Thigh shaper lunge ▶

(× 8 reps each leg)

Stand tall with tummy in tight and take a large step forward with right leg Ⓐ, bending both knees into a lunge with front knee in line with ankle Ⓑ. Straighten legs, then keep bending and straightening knees for 8 reps. When you have completed your reps on this side, step back and then step forward with other leg to repeat 8 lunges. Keep your body upright with tummy in tight throughout.

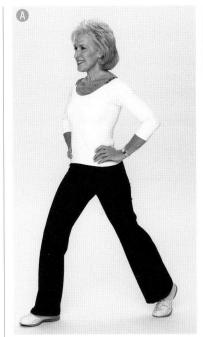
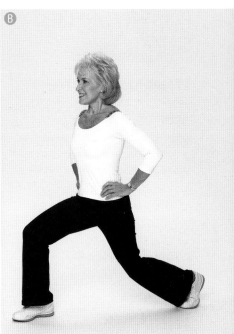

5 Top shoulder shaper ▶

(2 × 10 reps)

Stand tall with tummy in, feet apart and knees slightly bent. Hold arms by your sides with a weight or water bottle in each hand Ⓐ. Now breathe in and, as you breathe out, lift both arms out to shoulder height Ⓑ. Keep arms slightly bent and forward of body, with palms facing down. Do 10 reps, then rest before doing another set.

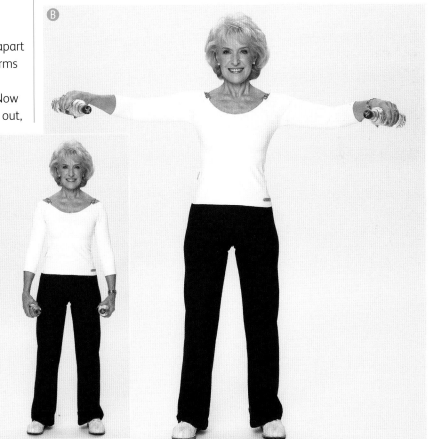

POST-WORKOUT STRETCHES

1 Front thigh stretch ▶

Lie on front, bend one knee and take hold of foot with hand on same side (or hold on to trouser leg or sock). Relax your upper body and gently press hip into floor to feel a stretch down front of thigh. Hold for 10 seconds, then change legs and repeat.

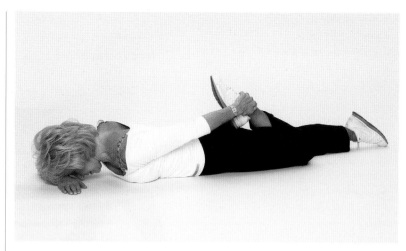

2 Tummy stretch ▶

Lie on front with arms at sides and elbows bent. Now prop up on your elbows, keeping hips in contact with floor, and lift chin forward slightly to feel a stretch in your tummy. Hold for 10 seconds, then release.

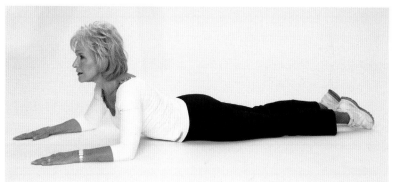

3 Outer thigh and hip stretch

Sit upright with legs straight out in front and bring left foot over right leg, placing foot flat on floor. Place left hand on floor for support and right hand across left knee. Use pressure of right arm to pull left leg further across body to feel a stretch in outer thigh and hip. Hold for 10 seconds, then change legs and repeat.

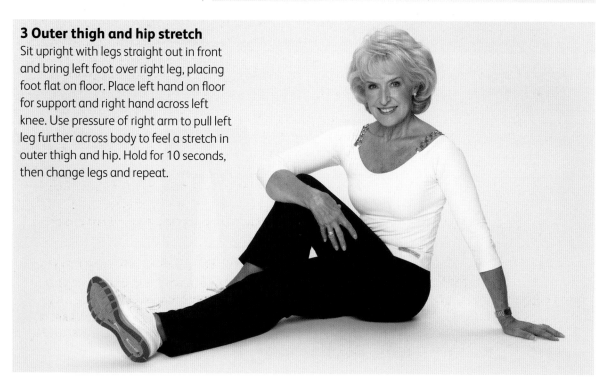

4 Chest stretch ▼

Sit upright and place both hands behind you on floor. Draw shoulders back to feel a stretch across chest, and hold for 10 seconds.

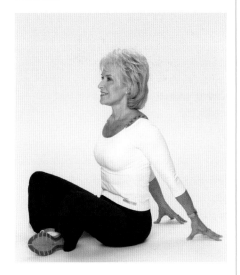

5 Shoulder stretch ▼

Sit upright with legs crossed and bring one arm across trunk at shoulder height. Use other arm to gently press on upper arm to stretch outside of shoulder. Hold for 10 seconds, then change arms and repeat.

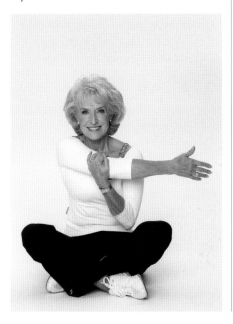

AEROBIC CHALLENGE

Go for a 20-minute brisk walk, then skip for 5 minutes (if you have a skipping rope). To finish, march on the spot for 2 minutes to cool down. Don't forget to do your stretches.

Exercise tip

You could increase your daily calorie output by as much as 200 extra calories just by making some small changes to your everyday routine. By using the stairs instead of the lift, parking your car further away or getting off the bus a stop earlier, walking to your colleague's desk to ask a question rather than phoning or e-mailing, standing up to make phone calls, taking a walk at lunchtime or going shopping and carrying the bags – all manner of little extras that mount up and burn extra calories.

MOTIVATIONAL THOUGHT FOR THE DAY

The fact that you have reached this exciting stage of your weight loss journey is very significant. The first two weeks were tough, but you managed. You are now five days into the second phase of this Amazing Inch Loss Plan and, despite having a couple of hundred extra calories to spend each day, your body is now in serious fat-burning mode. Your daily activity is being fuelled entirely from your fat stores and all the calories you are eating are being spent by your body to keep it functioning healthily.

Your body is being given five-star fuel, because everything you are eating is healthy, and your body is happy because it is in training to become fitter and to function at optimum efficiency. Our bodies were not designed to spend most of the day sitting behind a desk, in front of a computer, a steering wheel or a television. Our ancestors walked everywhere and spent most of the day outside, tending the land and growing their own food.

Should you get any hunger pangs, look upon this as a sign that your body is in calorie-deficit and you are getting slimmer by the day! If you feel really hungry between meals, have a low-calorie drink and nibble on some chopped vegetables. I know these are not as exciting as a packet of crisps but at least they won't make you fat.

Day 20

The exercises are becoming much more challenging now. Please try your best to do them, but if you find any of them too hard, just go back to the easier versions that you did a few days ago and then progress at a level that you feel is right for you. When you reach the end of the 28-day programme, I suggest you return to Day 14 and repeat the last two weeks of the exercise programme again, substituting the advanced versions of the individual toning exercises. If you are able to do them every day you will be astonished at how fast you will progress. But it's a myth to think that you have to be an exercise junkie to have a good body. Absolutely not. Once you have lost your unwanted weight, you can keep in great shape by doing a variety of exercises on a fairly regular basis.

Today's toning exercises work the abdominals, back and shoulders and hips. Once you master these more challenging moves, you will be able to work your muscles very effectively in a short period of time.

MENU

Breakfast
- Mix 100g 0% fat Greek yogurt with 1 blue Portion Pot® (40g) muesli and a little semi-skimmed milk from allowance to moisten. Add a little Silver Spoon Half Spoon to sweeten to taste. Leave to soak overnight in the refrigerator for best results. Serve chilled ☑

Mid-morning power snack
- 100g fresh pineapple ☑

Lunch
- Tuna or Chicken Pasta Salad: 1 red Portion Pot® (110g cooked weight) pasta shapes mixed with either 50g drained canned tuna (in brine) or 30g chopped cooked chicken breast, plus unlimited chopped peppers, red onion, cucumber, tomato and celery and 2 tsps Hellmann's Extra Light Mayonnaise or low-fat thousand island dressing
OR
- Any pre-packed sandwich (max. 300 kcal and 5% fat) ☑

Mid-afternoon power snack
- 20g low-fat cheese (max. 5% fat) plus 5 cherry tomatoes ☑

Dinner
- 150g tuna steak, grilled, served with 1 blue Portion Pot® (50g uncooked weight) couscous (any flavour, e.g. see Ainsley Harriott range) plus 1 blue Portion Pot® (75g) tomato salsa and a large salad
OR
- Roasted Pepper Pasta (see recipe, p.219) served with a large salad and low-fat dressing ☑

Dessert
- Eton Mess: Break up 1 Marks & Spencer meringue basket and mix with 1 tbsp 0% fat Greek yogurt and 1 large strawberry, chopped ☑

Alcohol or high-fat treat
- 75ml Martini Rosso plus a low-calorie mixer
OR
- 2 Galaxy Mini Eggs ☑

WARM-UP

Pretend skipping

Imagine you are holding a skipping rope. Begin a small bounce on the spot as you pretend to turn the rope. You can turn around in a circle and even do some fancy arm work such as figure 8s!

FIVE-MINUTE TONE-UP

1 Front shoulder shaper ▶

(3 × 10 reps)
Stand tall with back straight and hold a weight or water bottle in each hand, with backs of hands facing forward Ⓐ. Now breathe in and, as you breathe out, lift arms in front to shoulder height, keeping your shoulders down, head up and elbows slightly bent Ⓑ. Lower again slowly, and repeat. Do 10 reps, then rest before doing another 2 sets.

2 Waist shaper ▶

(2 × 8 reps each side)
Still holding weights or water bottles, bring both arms in front at shoulder height Ⓐ. Now pull left elbow back, bending arm and keeping it at shoulder height, with shoulders down and relaxed Ⓑ. Keep watching elbow so your head turns as well and keep hips facing front, with knees slightly bent. Do 8 reps to same side, then change sides and repeat. Rest before doing another set.

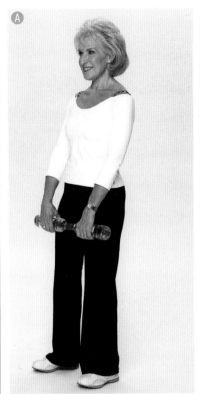

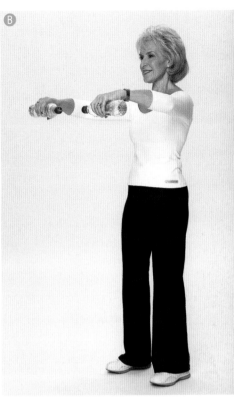

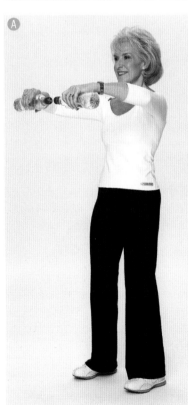

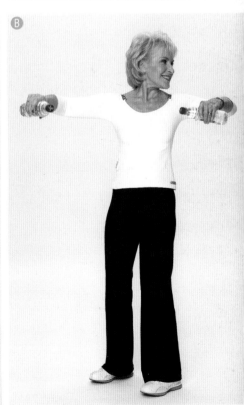

3 Advanced bottom shaper ▶

(2 × 8 reps alternate legs)
Lie on back with knees bent, feet together and arms by sides Ⓐ. Now breathe in and, as you breathe out, lift hips off floor without arching your back or coming up too high and, at same time, lift one leg to straighten it, keeping knees firmly together Ⓑ. Slowly lower hips and leg, then lift hips and other leg. Keep changing legs for 8 reps, then rest before doing another set.

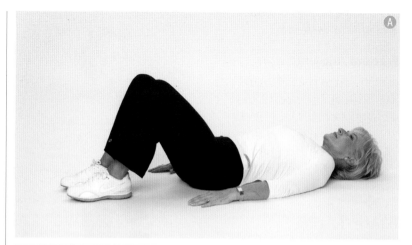

4 Tummy flattener ▼

(× 4 reps)
Lie on front and take a breath in. As you breathe out, pull tummy in very tight and lift trunk off the floor, propping yourself up on forearms and knees. Keep shoulders down and elbows directly under shoulders. Breathe normally and hold for about 10 seconds, then release. Do 4 reps.

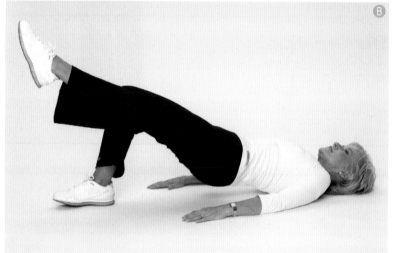

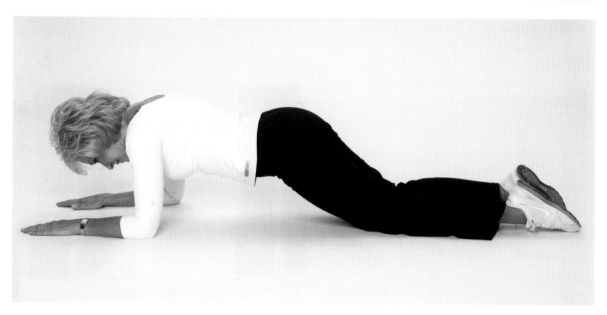

5 Posture improver and ▶ back strengthener

(2 × 8 reps)

Lie on front with arms by sides Ⓐ. Breathe out as you pull shoulders up and away from floor Ⓑ, then lift head off floor but keep looking down, with head in line with spine Ⓒ. Hold for 2 seconds, then breathe in and lower slowly. Do 8 reps, then rest before doing another set.

POST-WORKOUT STRETCHES

1 Tummy stretch ▼

Lie on front with arms at sides and elbows bent. Now prop up on your elbows, keeping hips in contact with floor, and lift chin forward slightly to feel a stretch in your tummy. Hold for 10 seconds, then release.

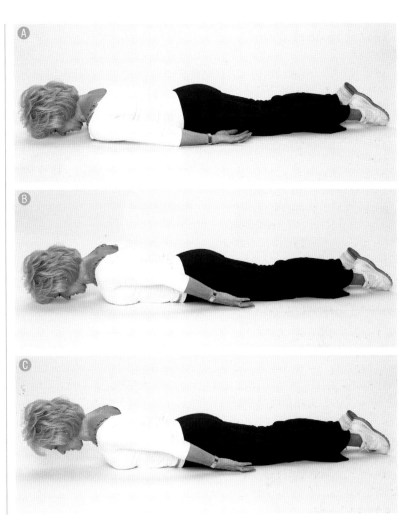

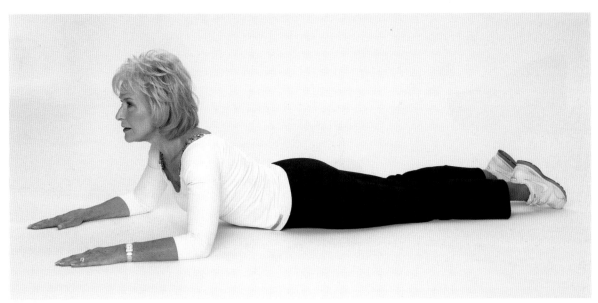

2 Front thigh stretch

Lie on front, bend one knee and take hold of foot with hand on same side (or hold on to trouser leg or sock). Relax your upper body and gently press hip into floor to feel a stretch down front of thigh.
Hold for 10 seconds, then change legs and repeat.

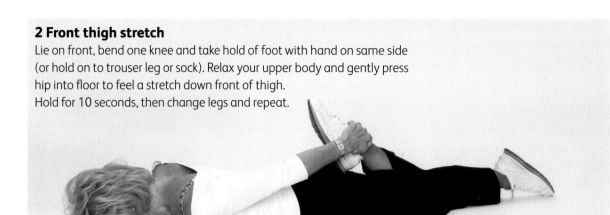

3 Waist stretch ▶

Sit up tall with legs crossed, then lift right arm and lean over to left side, keeping both hips on floor and without leaning forward or back. Hold for 10 seconds, then change sides and repeat.

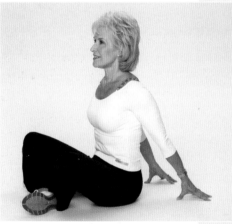

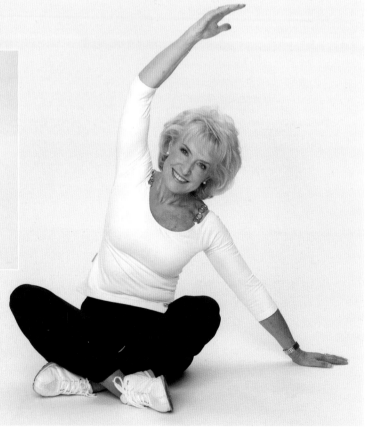

4 Chest stretch ▲

Still sitting upright, place both hands behind you on floor. Draw shoulders back to feel a stretch across chest, and hold for 10 seconds.

5 Back thigh stretch ▶

Sit upright with one leg straight out in front and the other bent. Place hands on floor at either side of straight leg and lean forward from hips to feel a stretch in back of thigh. Hold for 10 seconds, then try to lean a little further forward for another 10 seconds. Change legs and repeat.

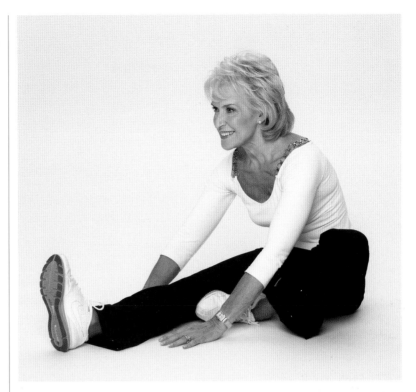

AEROBIC CHALLENGE

Work out energetically to a fitness DVD for 30 minutes or go for a 30-minute brisk walk.

Exercise tip

Next time you arrange to meet friends socially, why not suggest doing something active like ten pin bowling or ice skating or dancing. They are all great fun and much healthier than just sitting down eating and drinking all evening.

MOTIVATIONAL THOUGHT FOR THE DAY

Eating is an enjoyable habit but sometimes we can drift back into the old habits that made us overweight in the first place. We all have our favourite foods and it's fine to eat them occasionally, but only if we can trust ourselves not to eat them every day.

Eating big portions is another habit we can fall into. It is easy to convince ourselves that we are eating the correct amount of food, and staying within our daily calorie allowance, but often we are deceiving ourselves. Studies have shown that people tend to underestimate the quantity of food they eat and overestimate how active they are. That's why following a programme like the one in this book, where the calories are controlled and the exercises are specific, is so effective. So weigh out your portions (or use my Portion Pots®) to avoid disappointment on the scales. If you allow yourself that extra shake of cereal from the packet, that extra half tablespoon of boiled rice and curry and that extra glass of wine or orange juice, it really can affect your progress. So, in the run up to the last few days on this plan, make a massive effort to stick to the quantities given and to do the recommended activities. You will be grateful in the long run when you see the benefits.

Day 21

This is the final day of week three and it's your third weigh-in day tomorrow, so it's crucial you try to achieve as positive a response as possible on the scales. Be strict with your portion sizes, weighing out or measuring all your servings of food. Try to keep busy today so your mind is fully occupied and you are not constantly thinking about food. I also recommend you don't have any alcohol today as it can make you dehydrated and cause you to drink extra fluid to compensate, though I am in no way suggesting that you cut back on fluids. It is really important that you stay hydrated. You want to lose fat, not water.

Today is an aerobic day so there are no toning exercises, but aim to do as much aerobic activity as you can fit into your schedule as I really want you to keep moving as much as possible and burn lots of calories. Really go for it today.

MENU

Breakfast
■ 2 turkey rashers and 1 low-fat beef or pork sausage (max. 5% fat), grilled or dry-fried, served with 1 × 200g can tomatoes boiled until reduced and 100g grilled mushrooms **P**
OR
■ 2 Quorn sausages, grilled, served with 1 × 400g can tomatoes boiled until reduced, plus 50g grilled mushrooms **V**

Mid-morning power snack
■ 1 × 200g slice melon (weighed without skin) **V**

Lunch
■ Large mixed salad plus 1 smoked mackerel fillet or 1 × 125g can sardines or salmon (not in oil), served with 2 tsps Hellmann's Extra Light Mayonnaise or other low-fat dressing of your choice. Plus 1 pear or orange **P**
OR
■ Chicken, Mushroom and Lemon Soup (see recipe, p.210) served with a small wholegrain roll (max. 150 kcal). Plus 1 pear or orange

Mid-afternoon power snack
■ 150g strawberries **V**

Dinner
■ 100g lean roast beef, thinly sliced, served with 100g dry-roasted potatoes and 200g other vegetables of your choice (excluding potatoes), plus low-fat gravy and 1 tsp horseradish sauce
OR
■ Sweet and Sour Quorn: Dry-fry ½ pack (175g) of Quorn Chicken Style Pieces with ½ chopped onion, ½ chopped red and green pepper, 5 button mushrooms, halved, 1 chopped celery stick, 1 small courgette, halved and chopped, ½ pack of fresh (or 1 whole can) beansprouts. Do not overcook. Add 1 yellow Portion Pot® (125ml) Uncle Ben's Sweet & Sour Light sauce and heat through before serving **V** **P**
Plus 1 low-fat yogurt (max. 100 kcal and 5% fat) in addition to dessert below

Dessert
■ 1 Asda Good For You Lemon Slice **V**

Alcohol or high-fat treat
■ 300ml (½ pint) Guinness
OR
■ 1 Thorntons Mini Caramel Shortcake **V**

WARM-UP

March on spot with shoulder rolls

Stand tall and march on the spot for a total of 2 minutes. For every 4 steps, do a full shoulder roll, pulling shoulders forward, up, back and down.

AEROBIC CHALLENGE

Try and work out for an hour today. Salsacise, aerobics, a class, swimming energetically, working out to a DVD, using cardio equipment at the gym – they all use extra calories and they all burn fat. Drink plenty of water before, during and after your workout.

POST-AEROBIC STRETCHES

1 Calf stretch ▶

Place one foot in front of the other, with both feet pointing forward (hold on to a wall or sturdy surface for support if you wish). Bend front knee in line with ankle and keep back leg straight with heel pressing down. Lean further forward to feel a stretch in calf of back leg and hold for 10 seconds. Do the lower calf stretch (exercise 2, p.148) before changing legs.

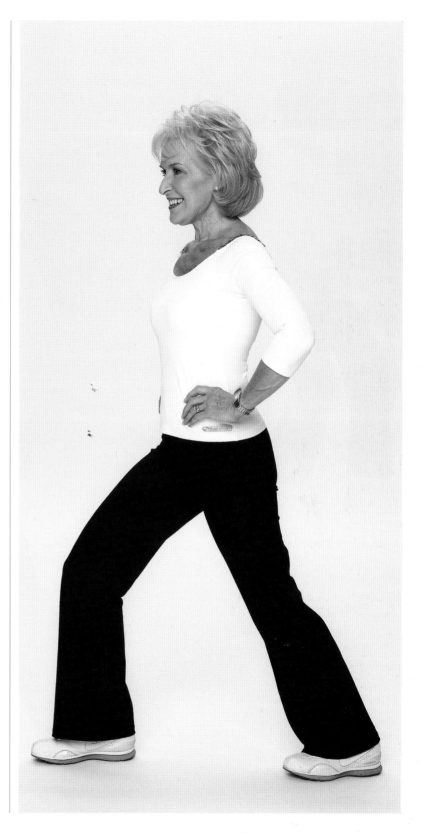

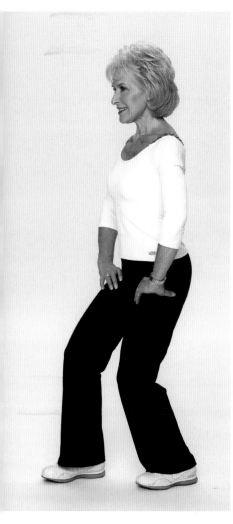

2 Lower calf stretch ▲

Bring your back foot half a step in
and bend both knees with feet still
pointing forward. Keep both heels
on floor and your body upright as
you look straight ahead and hold
for 10 seconds. Change legs and
repeat both calf stretches.

3 Back thigh stretch ▶

Straighten your front leg and keep
your back leg bent. With spine
straight, lean forward slightly to
feel a stretch in back thigh of
straight leg. Hold for 10 seconds,
then change legs and repeat.

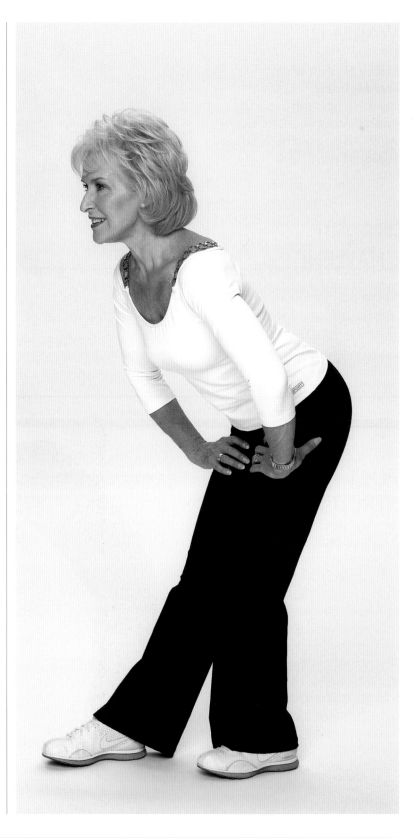

4 Front of hip stretch ▶

Bend front leg and lift heel of back foot. With your weight equally distributed between both legs, trunk upright and tummy in, press pelvis forward to feel a stretch at top of hip. Hold for 10 seconds, then change legs and repeat.

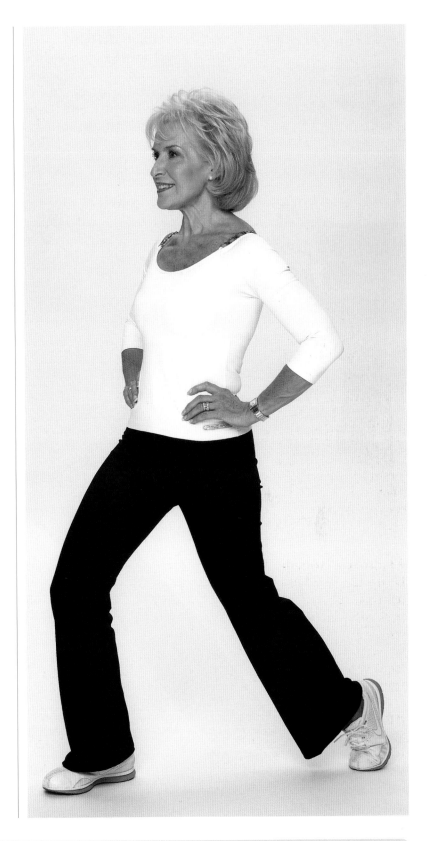

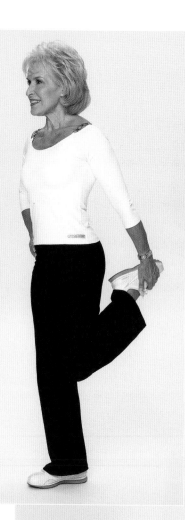

◀ 5 Front thigh stretch

Stand upright and take hold of one ankle with hand (place other hand on wall or back of chair for support if necessary). Bring knees in line with each other and keep supporting leg slightly bent. Gently push hip of raised leg forward to stretch front of thigh. Hold stretch for 10 seconds, then change legs and repeat.

6 Inner thigh stretch ▶

Stand tall and take legs out wide. Bend one knee in line with ankle, keeping other leg straight with foot pointing forward, to feel a stretch in inner thigh of straight leg. Hold for 10 seconds, then change legs and repeat.

Washing the car is an excellent workout. It involves quite a lot of energy and strength to clean and polish the paintwork before it dries too quickly to prevent those ugly smears. See your car washing as a workout and do it more often.

MOTIVATIONAL THOUGHT FOR THE DAY

Try to make a special effort with your appearance today and wear something that shows you have lost weight. Put on some make-up, style your hair carefully and wear some pretty jewellery.

If someone compliments you on your appearance, accept the compliment with good grace. Thank the person and say: 'That's really encouraging. I am trying very hard to lose weight at the moment.' Often when someone pays us a compliment we get embarrassed and throw it back at them by saying something like: 'Well yes, I've lost a bit, but I'm still huge.' You can be pretty sure that the person who made the kind comment won't venture there again!

So, make a conscious decision that if someone does make a flattering comment you will enjoy it and be ready with your gracious response.

Day 22

Today is your third weighing and measuring day. This third weigh-in is perhaps the hardest to face, as you have increased your calories a little over the last week and your body has now got used to eating fewer calories than it was receiving up to three weeks ago. As a result, you may not see the same level of weight loss on the scales as you did at the end of week two. This is to be expected, so please don't be discouraged.

You are probably finding you get a bit hungry more often – but remember, this is great news as it shows your body is having to draw on your energy stores of fat distributed around your body to make up the shortfall. Also, you might be finding that your energy levels are flagging a little, as your body is now in full fat-burning mode. I can only promise you that it will get easier and you only have one week to go at this lower calorie level. I've given you a rest day from aerobic exercise today, and the five-minute tone-up is quick to do and doesn't use too much energy, yet it is extremely effective. Today's exercises work the abdominals and back, the outer thighs, and the chest and underarm muscles. Just stick with it and trust me that the results in a week's time will be worth it.

MENU

Breakfast
- 2 Weetabix served with milk from allowance and 2 tsps sugar or 1 mini banana ✓

Mid-morning power snack
- 1 small apple ✓

Lunch
- 1 × 40g granary baguette spread with 20g Philadelphia Extra Light soft cheese then topped with 25g wafer thin ham or Quorn Deli Ham Style, 1 sliced tomato and mustard to taste, plus a small side salad ✓

Mid-afternoon power snack
- 1 Rakusen's cracker topped with 1 × 20g triangle Laughing Cow Extra Light soft cheese, plus 5 cherry tomatoes

Dinner
- Fish Pie: Place 50g each of fresh salmon, cod and shelled uncooked prawns in a small ovenproof dish and cover with ⅓ can Batchelors Low Fat Condensed Mushroom Soup, top with mashed potato (made by boiling 115g old potatoes then mashing with milk from allowance and seasoning well). Place in the oven and bake at 200C, 400F, Gas Mark 6 for 30 minutes or until the potato is browned on top. Serve with unlimited carrots and broccoli P
OR
- Quorn and Rice Bake (see recipe, p.220) served with unlimited vegetables (excluding potatoes) ✓

Dessert
- 1 × 70g pot Marks & Spencer Count On Us Raspberry Mousse

Alcohol or high-fat treat
- 1 yellow Portion Pot® (125ml) red or white wine
OR
- 1 McVitie's Belgian Chocolate Chunk Boaster ✓

WARM-UP

Twisted canoeing

Stand tall and bring both arms overhead with tummy in. Now drop both arms to one side as you bend your knees and hips, then come up and repeat, dropping your arms to the other side. Keep going for 1 minute.

FIVE-MINUTE TONE-UP

1 Tummy curl with ▶ extra lift

(✕ 6 reps)

Lie on back with knees bent, feet flat on floor and hands behind head. Pull tummy in tight and, as you breathe out, lift head and shoulders off floor Ⓐ. Breathe in and bring both arms forward Ⓑ and, as you breathe out, lift further Ⓒ, keeping chin off chest and holding tummy in throughout. Slowly lower again and repeat. Do 6 reps.

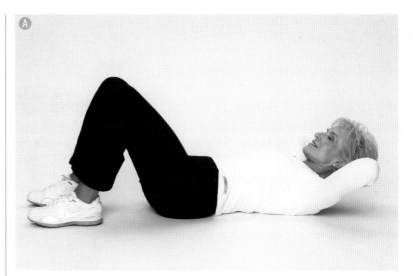

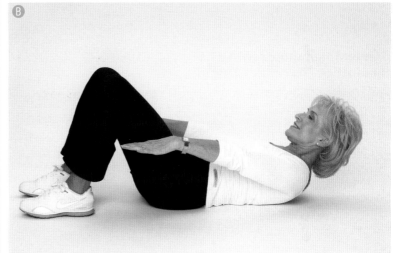

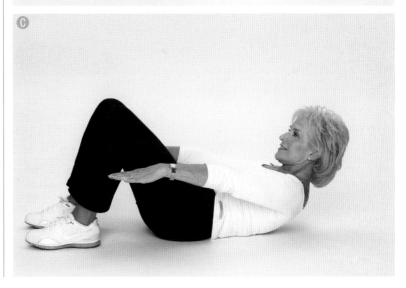

2 Advanced waist twist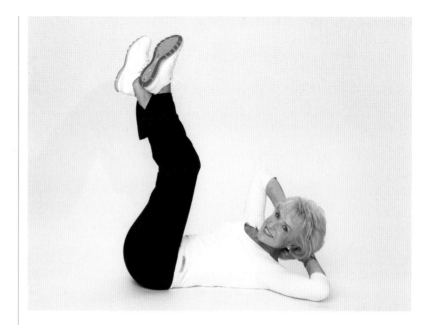

(2 × 12 alternate sides)

Lie on back with hands behind head, feet off floor and ankles crossed. Breathe in and, as you breathe out, pull tummy in tight and lift head and shoulders off floor, bringing right shoulder up towards left thigh. Lower again, then come up to other side. Keep alternating sides for 12 reps, then rest before repeating another set.

3 Outer thigh shaper with three-stage lift

(× 8 reps each leg)

Lie on side, bend bottom leg up to 90 degrees and push top leg out straight in line with hip, foot flexed, and hold a weight on thigh. Pull tummy in to hold trunk still, then lift top leg slightly and pause Ⓐ. Now lift leg again to mid range and pause Ⓑ, then lift to top of range and pause Ⓒ, keeping hips stacked. Lower under control in one movement, and repeat. Do 8 reps on one leg, then roll over and repeat on other leg.

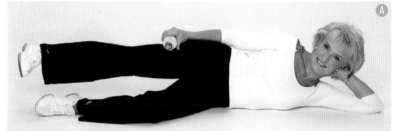

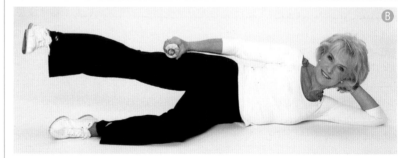

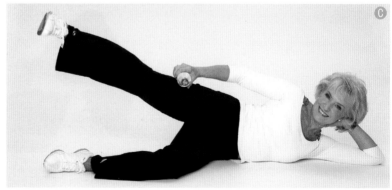

4 Spine stabiliser ▶

(× 8 reps alternate sides)
Come onto hands and knees
with knees under hips and your
shoulders over your wrists. Now
slide right hand and left foot along
the floor until leg and arm are as
straight as possible Ⓐ. Hold tummy
in tight, then lift leg and arm off
floor in line with the trunk Ⓑ. Hold
for 3 seconds, then release, and
repeat on other side. Do 8 reps,
changing sides each time.

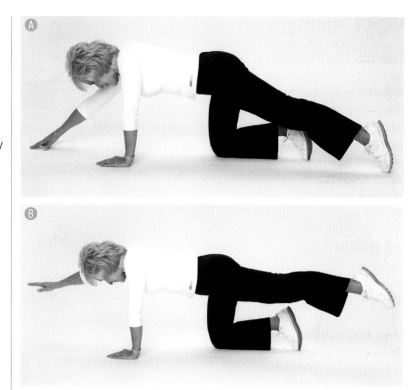

5 Chest and underarm ▶ toner

(2 × 12 reps)
Start on hands and knees, with
hands under shoulders and your
knees under hips, then move knees
further back and pull tummy in Ⓐ.
Breathe in as you lower upper body
towards floor, bending elbows
outward and leading with chest Ⓑ.
Breathe out as you push up again
without locking elbows. Do 12 reps,
then rest and build up to another
set.

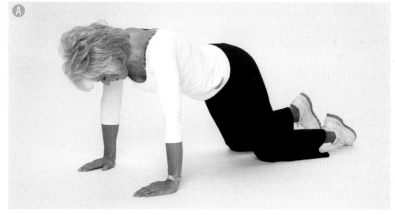

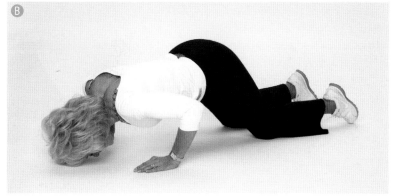

POST-WORKOUT STRETCHES

1 Tummy stretch ▶

Lie on front with arms at sides and elbows bent. Now prop up on your elbows, keeping hips in contact with floor, and lift your chin forward slightly to feel a stretch in your tummy. Hold for 10 seconds, then release.

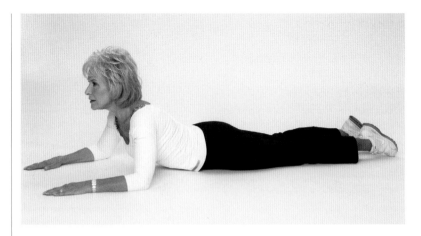

2 Back stretch ▶

Come up onto your hands and knees and, as you pull your tummy in, arch your spine up towards the ceiling, letting your head drop down. Hold for 10 seconds, then release.

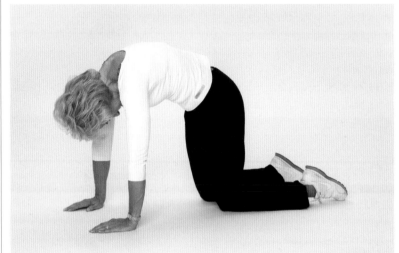

3 Outer thigh and hip ▶ stretch

Sit upright with legs straight out in front and bring left foot over right leg, placing foot flat on floor. Place left hand on floor for support and right hand across left knee. Use pressure of right arm to pull left leg further across body to feel a stretch in outer thigh and hip. Hold for 10 seconds, then change legs and repeat.

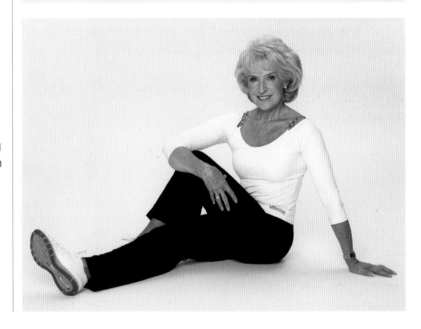

4 Chest stretch ▶

Sit upright with legs crossed and place both hands behind you on floor. Draw shoulders back to feel a stretch across chest, and hold for 10 seconds.

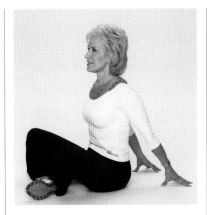

5 Waist stretch ▶

Still sitting up tall with legs crossed, lift right arm and lean over to left side, keeping both hips on floor and without leaning forward or back. Hold for 10 seconds, then change sides and repeat.

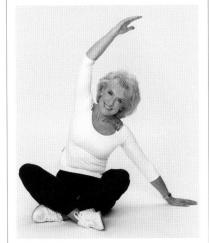

6 Underarm stretch ▶

Place right hand behind right shoulder. Press left hand on right underarm to push right hand further down your back. Keep your head up and look straight ahead. Hold for 10 seconds, then change arms and repeat.

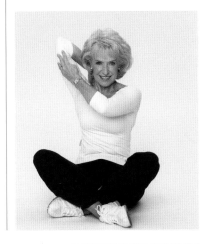

Exercise tip

Try balancing on one leg when you are cleaning your teeth or talking on the phone. This might sound odd, but it will help to improve your balance as well as your posture. Balance is something we can learn at any age and it helps us to stay safe as we are less likely to fall over.

MOTIVATIONAL THOUGHT FOR THE DAY

When you got on the scales this morning, if you found you hadn't lost the half stone you felt you deserved to have lost this week because you have been so good, don't despair. Measure yourself and see for yourself that lots of inches have in fact disappeared this week and that is what matters. You are getting slimmer. People are noticing and your clothes are looser.

The mid-morning and mid-afternoon power snacks are there to help you stave off hunger pangs, so make sure you eat them. It's important that you don't eat less food than is recommended in the eating plan. And are you drinking enough fluids? Sometimes our energy levels can plummet if we get dehydrated, so drink plenty of water, weak tea or low-calorie drinks to keep your fluid levels adequately topped up.

Enjoy your toning exercises today. As your muscles are now stronger, you will be able to do these more advanced moves and reap the benefits to your body shape. And the aerobic challenge will help you to burn more body fat, so do your best to fit it in. You are winning the weight loss battle and the rewards are huge.

Day 23

Now you are well into week four, take time to appreciate your monumental achievements so far. Your body is getting used to eating healthier food, doing lots of different exercises and will be feeling slimmer and fitter. What are the things you have noticed most? Are you finding it easier to fit into the bath? Do you no longer get so out of breath when you go upstairs? Are your clothes feeling looser and more comfortable rather than feeling as if they are 'strangling' you? No doubt you are experiencing enormous benefits all round.

The daily exercises are becoming increasingly challenging as each day progresses, so listen to your body and only do what you feel you can manage. Today we are using a chair again and the workout includes exercises for the stomach, backside, inner and front thighs as well as the underarms. The harder the exercises become, the more effective they will be at strengthening and shaping your muscles. And the stronger your muscles, the greater the amount of fat that will be burnt in them when you do your aerobic exercises. Be encouraged. You are really doing the business now and your body is undergoing a significant transformation.

MENU

Breakfast
- ½ fresh grapefruit plus 2 medium-sized boiled eggs ☑ P

Mid-morning power snack
- 1 blue Portion Pot® (75g) tomato salsa, plus 1 carrot, 1 celery stick and 1 × 5cm piece cucumber sliced into crudités ☑

Lunch
- Chicken and Rice Salad: 80g (cooked weight) boiled basmati rice mixed with 60g cooked chopped chicken breast (no skin), chopped peppers, red onion, mushrooms, celery and 1 tbsp sweetcorn kernels. Season with freshly ground black pepper and soy sauce or fat-free dressing of your choice
OR
- Singapore Noodles with Prawns (see recipe, p.218) plus a crisp salad

Mid-afternoon power snack
- 1 fat-free yogurt (max. 50 kcal) ☑

Dinner
- Baked Liver and Onions: Place 150g calves' liver in an ovenproof dish with 1 sliced onion. Cover with foil and cook in a moderate oven (180C, 350F, Gas Mark 4) for 15–20 minutes until lightly cooked. Make some low-fat gravy with gravy powder and add to the liver and onion. Serve with 1 yellow Portion Pot® (100g) mashed potato and other vegetables of your choice
OR
- Cheesy Cottage Pie (see recipe, p.214)

Dessert
- Tropical Sorbet (see recipe, p.222) ☑

Alcohol or high-fat treat
- 300ml (½ pint) lager or beer
OR
- 1 Kellogg's Coco Pops Cereal & Milk Bar ☑

WARM-UP

Ski swings

Stand tall and lift both arms overhead, pulling your tummy in. Now swing arms down and past your thighs as you bend your knees and hips. Keep your back straight and keep looking forward. Come up again and repeat ski swings for 1 minute.

FIVE-MINUTE TONE-UP

1 Three-stage chair squat ▶

(2 × 6 reps)
Stand in front of a sturdy chair with feet hip width apart and a weight in each hand Ⓐ. Pull tummy in tight, then bend hips back just a little and pause Ⓑ. Hold for just a second, then lower hips a little further and pause Ⓒ before lowering hips further so they just touch chair seat Ⓓ. Come up again in one movement. Do 6 reps, then rest before doing another set.

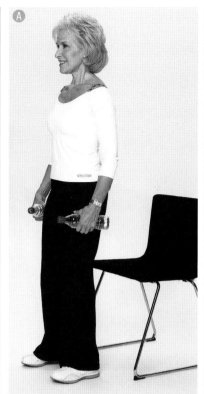

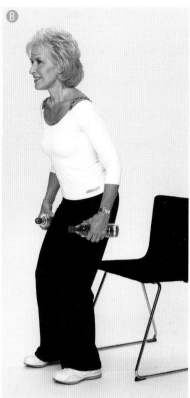

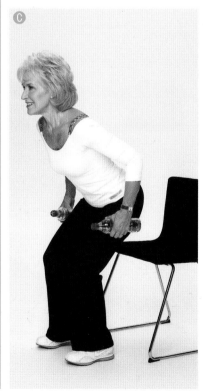

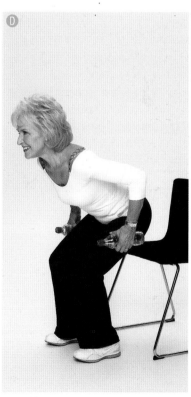

2 Advanced underarm toner ▶

(2 × 8 reps)

Start with both hands resting on the edge of chair seat and hips close to chair Ⓐ. Pull tummy in tight and bend the elbows, taking hips towards floor Ⓑ. Push back up again, keeping your shoulders down and your head up. Do 8 reps, then build up to another set

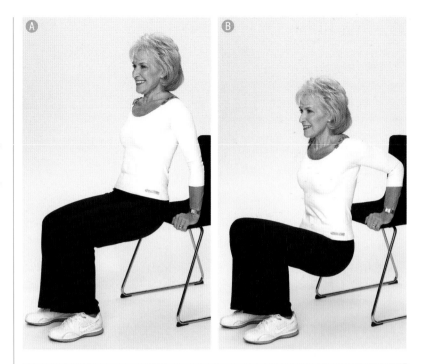

3 Advanced bottom toner ▶

(2 × 8 reps)

Lie on back with arms by sides, heels resting on chair seat and legs slightly bent Ⓐ. Breathe in and, as you breathe out, lift hips off floor, holding your tummy in and keeping neck and shoulders relaxed Ⓑ. Slowly lower hips again, and repeat. Do 8 reps, then rest before doing another set.

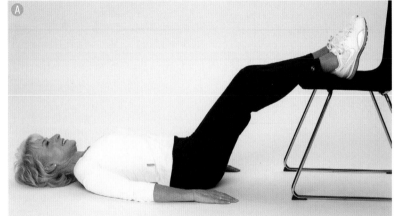

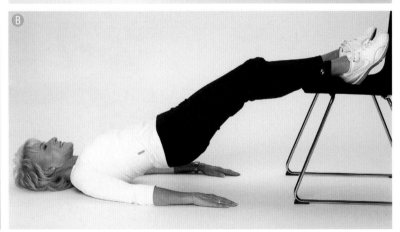

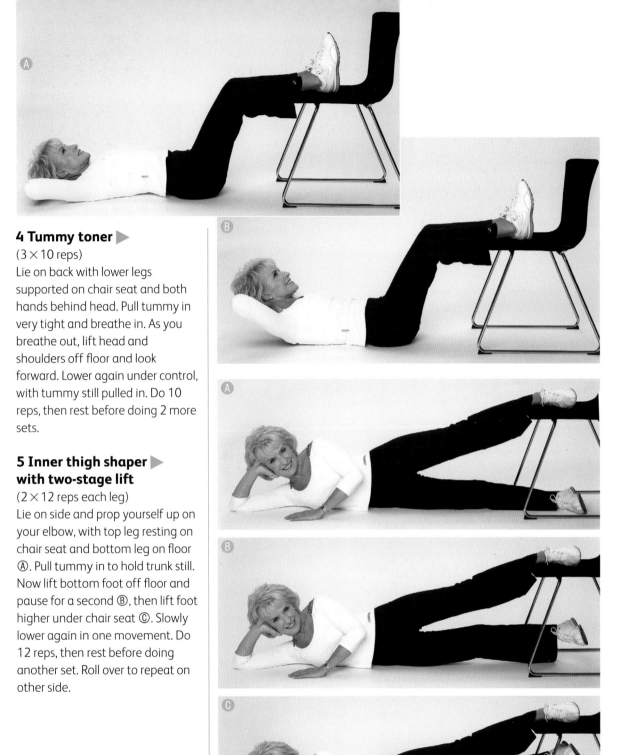

4 Tummy toner ▶

(3 × 10 reps)

Lie on back with lower legs supported on chair seat and both hands behind head. Pull tummy in very tight and breathe in. As you breathe out, lift head and shoulders off floor and look forward. Lower again under control, with tummy still pulled in. Do 10 reps, then rest before doing 2 more sets.

5 Inner thigh shaper ▶ with two-stage lift

(2 × 12 reps each leg)

Lie on side and prop yourself up on your elbow, with top leg resting on chair seat and bottom leg on floor Ⓐ. Pull tummy in to hold trunk still. Now lift bottom foot off floor and pause for a second Ⓑ, then lift foot higher under chair seat Ⓒ. Slowly lower again in one movement. Do 12 reps, then rest before doing another set. Roll over to repeat on other side.

POST-WORKOUT STRETCHES

1 Back thigh stretch ▶

Sit on front third of chair seat and straighten left leg
with both hands resting on thigh. Now, keeping your
back straight and looking forward, lean forward from
hips to feel a stretch in back of thigh. Hold for 10
seconds, then change legs and repeat.

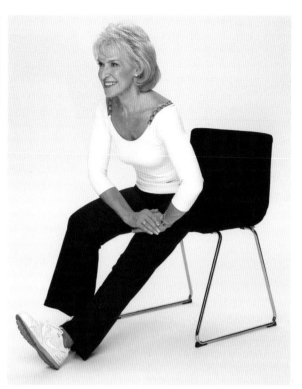

2 Inner thigh stretch ▼

Still sitting on chair, bend knees and bring feet
together, then press hands on inside of thighs to push
knees outward but keeping feet in contact with each
other. Hold stretch for 10 seconds, then release.

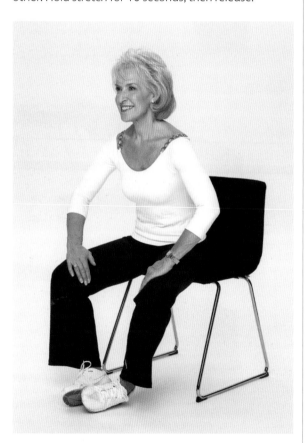

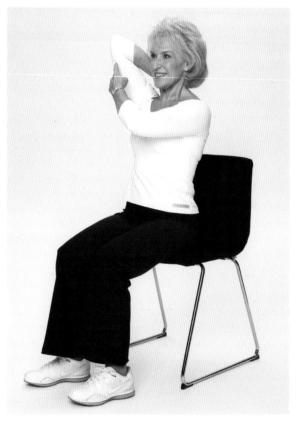

3 Underarm stretch ▶

Sitting with knees bent, place right hand behind
shoulder. Press left hand on right underarm to push
hand further down your back. Keep your head up and
look straight ahead. Hold stretch for 10 seconds, then
change arms and repeat.

4 Waist stretch ▶

Place right hand on chair for support. Lift left arm and bend to right without leaning forward or back and keeping both hips firmly on seat of chair, to feel a stretch down left side. Hold for 10 seconds, then change sides and repeat.

5 Front thigh stretch ▶▶

Stand and hold on to back of chair with right hand. Take left ankle in left hand (or hold trouser leg or sock) and bring knees in line with each other, then press left hip forward to feel a stretch down front of thigh. Hold for 10 seconds, then change legs and repeat.

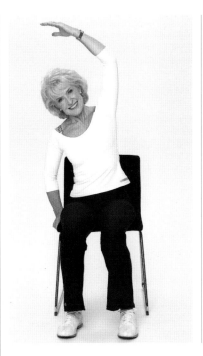
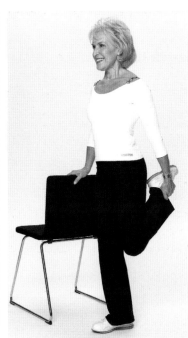

AEROBIC CHALLENGE

Work out at an aerobics class or to a fitness DVD for 40 minutes, or go for a 40-minute brisk walk, or walk up and down stairs 5 times consecutively and repeat 3 times throughout the day.

Exercise tip

If you have a small trampoline or any piece of home gym equipment, why not get it out of the loft or the garage, dust it off and have a go on it. Put on some lively music and bounce, pedal, row or run on it. Exercise can be monotonous sometimes and if we vary our activities, we are more likely to keep it up.

MOTIVATIONAL THOUGHT FOR THE DAY

If we are to succeed at anything – and that includes losing weight and getting fitter – it's crucial that we are motivated by the end goal, and the rewards that we enjoy along the way will help us to reach that goal.

Rewards are very motivating and at least 50 per cent of the pleasure is the 'looking forward to it' bit. So, decide what you would like as a reward for each stone you lose or for when your weight enters a new weight-bracket (such as getting to 12 stone-something from being 13 stone-something) and then decide on an ultimate reward for when you reach your goal weight.

If you have a generous and supportive partner, maybe they could sponsor you for each pound or stone you lose so that you can treat yourself to some lovely new clothes when you reach your goal. Or perhaps you dream of having a makeover or going to a health spa for a weekend or even just for a day. You choose, but discuss it with the family so that they know where you are aiming and they can encourage you and enjoy the journey with you.

Start planning a reward for your efforts this week, even if you don't actually receive the reward until some time in the future. If you have to wait, you can enjoy the looking-forward-to-it bit all the more!

Day 24

As you move towards the end of the 28-day programme, really step up your efforts with the exercise plan. The more challenging the exercises become, the more effective they will be.

Today's toning exercises work the abdominals, back and shoulders, and outer thighs. Try to perform them to the best of your ability and don't rush them, but feel the action of each muscle as it works hard. Focus on that feeling in the muscle to help maximise the effect of the exercise and also to make sure you are doing the exercise correctly. If you can't feel anything happening to the muscle, probably not much will be happening! So read the instructions for each exercise carefully and make sure your body position is accurate so you can enjoy the best possible benefits and results.

Your aerobic fitness should have improved significantly by now. Try to walk a bit faster and jog for longer if you can. If jogging proves too difficult for you, because of pressure on your knees or hips, then try power walking, which is just as effective providing you don't mind keeping going for a little longer to cover the same distance. Both jogging and power walking are fantastic fat burners.

MENU

Breakfast
■ 200g fresh fruit salad topped with 100g Total 2% fat Greek Yoghurt and 6 sultanas ☑

Mid-morning power snack
■ 10 cherry tomatoes, plus chunks of carrots, cucumber and green or red pepper ☑

Lunch
■ 1 bagel cut in half, spread with 20g Philadelphia Extra Light soft cheese then topped with 50g smoked salmon and freshly ground black pepper or chopped fresh dill
OR
■ 1 × 50g wholemeal pitta bread filled with 50g low-fat houmous and chopped mixed salad sprinkled with low-fat dressing of your choice ☑

Mid-afternoon power snack
■ 2 satsumas ☑

Dinner
■ Steak in Mushroom Sauce: Dry-fry 2 thin beef steaks (250g total) or 2 Quorn Peppered Steaks quickly on both sides. Remove from the pan and keep warm. Add 100g chestnut mushrooms to the pan and cook for 1 minute before adding 1 tsp Knorr Touch of Taste beef stock (or vegetarian alternative) and 75ml water. Bring the sauce to the boil and reduce by half. Remove from the heat and stir in ½ tbsp 3% fat yogurt. Transfer the steaks to serving plates and top with the mushroom sauce. Serve with green vegetables or salad ☑ ℗
OR
■ Chinese Chicken Kebabs (see recipe, p.211) served with 1 blue Portion Pot® (55g uncooked weight) or 1 red Portion Pot® (144g cooked weight) basmati rice per person

Dessert
■ 1 × 70g pot Marks & Spencer Count On Us Chocolate Mousse

Alcohol or high-fat treat
■ 50ml measure of port
OR
■ 1 Green & Black's Organic Chocolate Flapjack biscuit ☑

WARM-UP

Stair step-ups

Using a single step (such as bottom step of your stairs), step up and down for 2 minutes. Lead with the right leg for 1 minute, then pause and change to lead with the left leg. Make sure the whole foot makes contact on each step.

FIVE-MINUTE TONE-UP

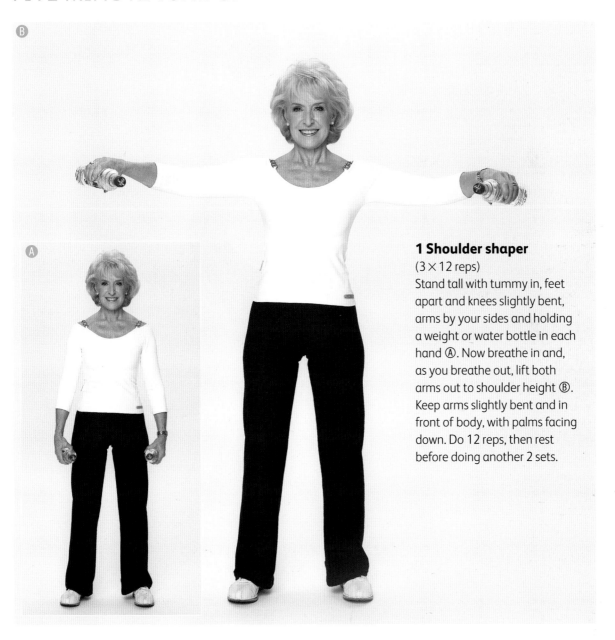

1 Shoulder shaper
(3 × 12 reps)
Stand tall with tummy in, feet apart and knees slightly bent, arms by your sides and holding a weight or water bottle in each hand Ⓐ. Now breathe in and, as you breathe out, lift both arms out to shoulder height Ⓑ. Keep arms slightly bent and in front of body, with palms facing down. Do 12 reps, then rest before doing another 2 sets.

2 Tummy crunch ▶

(2 × 8 reps)

Lie on back with legs raised and ankles crossed. Place both hands behind head and pull tummy in tight Ⓐ. Now breathe out as you lift head and shoulders off floor and, at same time, lift hips up slightly Ⓑ. Keep your chin off your chest and hold your tummy in throughout. Do 8 reps, then rest before doing another set.

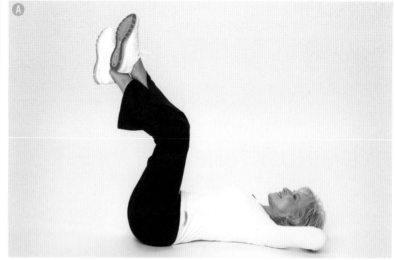

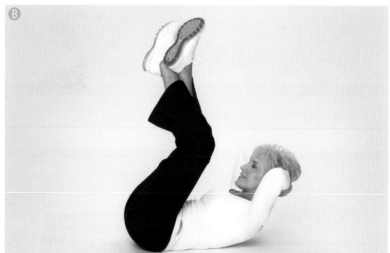

3 Advanced waist shaper ▶

(2 × 8 reps alternate sides)

Start in the same position as Exercise 2 and, as you breathe out and lift head and shoulders off floor, reach one arm up and across towards opposite foot. Slowly lower again, and repeat to other side. Keep changing sides for 8 reps, then rest before doing another set.

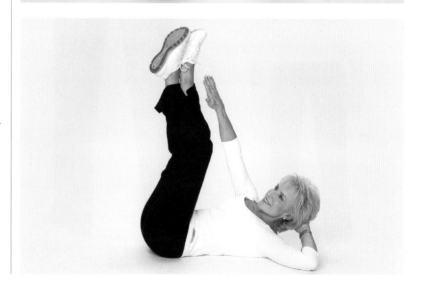

4 Outer thigh shaper ▶ with three-stage lift

(× 10 reps each leg)

Lie on side, bend bottom leg up to 90 degrees and push top leg out straight in line with hip, foot flexed, and hold a weight on thigh. Pull tummy in to hold trunk still, then lift top leg slightly and pause Ⓐ. Now lift leg again to mid range and pause Ⓑ, then lift to top of range and pause Ⓒ, keeping hips stacked. Lower under control in one movement, and repeat. Do 10 reps on one leg, then roll over and repeat on other leg.

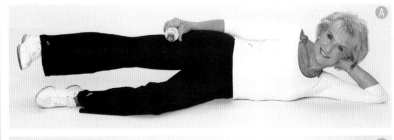

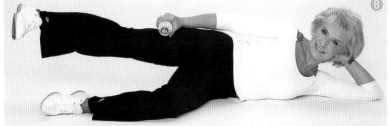

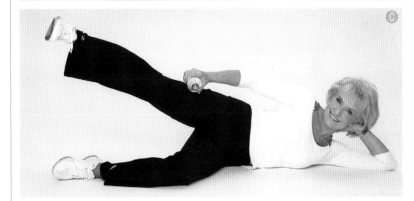

5 Posture improver and ▶ back strengthener

(2 × 6 reps)

Lie on front with arms by sides Ⓐ. Breathe out as you pull shoulders up and away from floor Ⓑ, then lift head off floor but keep looking down, with head in line with spine Ⓒ. Hold for 2 seconds, then breathe in and lower slowly. Do 6 reps, then rest before doing another set.

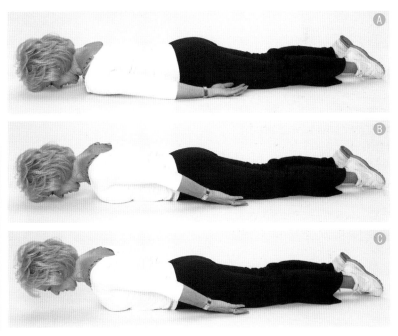

POST-WORKOUT STRETCHES

1 Tummy stretch ▶

Lie on front with arms at sides and elbows bent. Now prop up on your forearms, keeping hips in contact with floor, and lift your chin forward slightly to feel a stretch in your tummy. Hold for 10 seconds, then release.

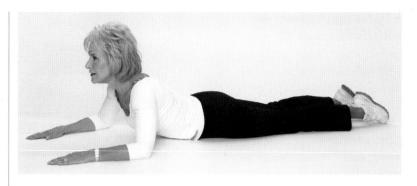

2 Back stretch ▶

Come up onto your hands and knees and, as you pull your tummy in, arch your spine up towards ceiling, letting your head drop down. Hold for 10 seconds, then release.

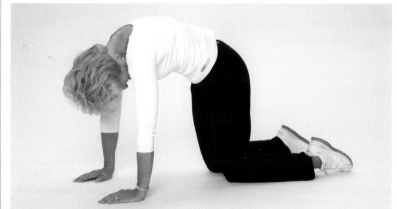

3 Waist stretch ▶

Lie on back with knees bent, feet flat on floor and place arms out at sides at shoulder height with palms down. Pull tummy in and gently roll knees to right side as you look at your left hand and feel a stretch in waist. Hold for 10 seconds, then roll over to other side and hold again.

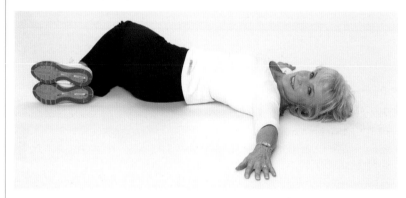

4 Outer thigh and hip ▶ stretch

Lie on back with knees bent, then place one ankle across other knee and let raised knee drop out to side. Stay there if you feel a strong stretch in outer thigh and hip and hold for 10 seconds. For a stronger stretch, lift other foot off floor, then bring knees closer to chest and hold for 10 seconds. Change legs and repeat.

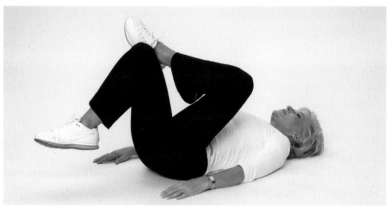

5 Shoulder stretch ▶

Sit upright with legs crossed and bring right arm across body at shoulder height. Use left arm to gently press on upper arm to stretch outside of shoulder. Hold for 10 seconds, then change arms and repeat.

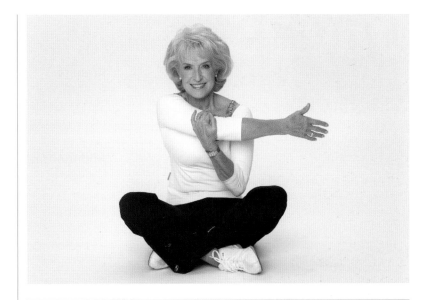

AEROBIC CHALLENGE

Go for a power walk and intersperse some jogging steps even if you manage only 20 or so. Try to keep going for 30 minutes.

Exercise tip

Did you know that dog walkers are on average a stone lighter than non-dog owners? Dog walking is a great way to burn extra calories. It works because the dog provides the purpose for the excursion and the motivation to put on your walking shoes. As one doctor told me: 'The NHS should provide everyone with a dog – it would transform their health!' If you don't have a dog of your own, maybe you could borrow one from a friend or neighbour?

MOTIVATIONAL THOUGHT FOR THE DAY

Just four days to go after today and then you can calculate how many calories you are allowed each day on the third phase of this Amazing Inch Loss Plan in order to continue to lose the rest of your unwanted weight. The heavier you are, the more calories you will be allowed and if you are young, you will be surprised at how many you can have.

As we get older we burn fewer calories, so we have to accept that we must eat less if we are to avoid weight gain. We tend not to be as active as we were in our twenties and so sometimes, thankfully, our appetite will decrease too. Mine certainly did as I reached my late fifties and early sixties and I now find that I can get halfway through a meal and my stomach says: 'That's it! I don't want any more.' I don't fight it. I'm just really glad that my appestat (the bit of our brain that tells us when we've eaten enough) is working at last!

Over the last three-and-a-half weeks you have re-educated your appetite, your palate and your eating habits, and the changes you have made will have turned your body into a highly efficient machine. Your blood pressure and your cholesterol levels will be healthier, your muscles will have become stronger and your organs – liver, kidneys, etc. – will feel like they've had a holiday as they won't have had to work so hard processing all the high-fat food you ate previously. By the end of this week you will have given your body the equivalent of a 50,000-mile service and it will be feeling terrific. Keep up your new healthy way of eating and your increased activity levels so you can allow the transformation to continue.

Day 25

Are you still sticking strictly to the diet? It's important that you still keep tabs on what you are eating and don't become too relaxed. Adding an extra slice of ham to your sandwich ('to finish off the packet'), or eating a couple of sweets offered by colleagues and finishing those leftovers on the children's plates are all pitfalls to which we can easily succumb, and the cumulative value of the extra calories in a day could easily be 500! Over a week that would amount to one pound of body fat and the spoiling of your weight loss progress. So be extra-vigilant over these last few days and be as active as you possibly can. 'Walk more, drive less' is this week's motto!

Today's toning exercises are even more challenging. Do try them, but if you find a particular exercise too tough, return to the previous exercise that you managed to complete satisfactorily for that part of the body. As you become fitter and stronger you will be able to progress to these advanced moves. Today we are working the stomach, back, backside, legs and shoulders. Do your best.

MENU

Breakfast
- ½ bagel (or 1 whole mini bagel) toasted, spread with 1 tsp fruit preserve, jam, honey or marmalade then topped with 50g 2% fat Total Greek Yoghurt ☑

Mid-morning power snack
- 1 kid's fun-size mini banana ☑

Lunch
- 75g cooked egg noodles tossed with unlimited beansprouts, spring onions, chopped peppers, fresh coriander and 75g flaked cooked salmon, served with soy sauce
OR
- Cheese and Marmite Sandwich: Spread 2 slices wholegrain bread with Marmite and fill with 40g low-fat cottage cheese ☑

Mid-afternoon power snack
- 1 kiwi fruit plus 5 seedless grapes ☑

Dinner
- Beef Fajitas: Dry-fry 120g sliced lean beef with ½ each sliced red and green pepper and ½ chopped red onion, then mix in 2 tsps fajita spice mix. Fill a low-fat tortilla wrap with the mixture and serve with 1 blue Portion Pot® (75g) tomato salsa and a large mixed salad tossed in oil-free dressing
OR
- Chicken Shaslik (see recipe, p.212) served with 1 blue Portion Pot® (55g uncooked weight) or 1 red Portion Pot® (144g cooked weight) basmati rice per person

Dessert
- 1 × 200g pot Müllerlight Wild Blueberry fat free yogurt

Alcohol or high-fat treat
- 1 blue Portion Pot® (80ml) dry sherry
OR
- 6 Cadbury Mini Eggs ☑

WARM-UP

March on spot with tummy pull-ins

Stand tall and march on the spot, letting the arms swing naturally. Every 10 steps, really pull your tummy in tight and then relax it for 10 steps.

FIVE-MINUTE TONE-UP

1 One-legged squat ▶

(2 × 6 reps each leg)
Stand tall with hands on hips or on back of a chair for support. Place right foot behind left ankle and pull tummy in to help you balance Ⓐ. Now bend left knee, pushing hips back Ⓑ. Come up again without locking knee of supporting leg. Do 6 reps slowly, then change legs and repeat. Rest before doing another set.

> If balancing on one leg is too difficult, keep both feet on floor.

2 Front shoulder shaper ▶

(3 × 12 reps)
Stand tall with back straight and hold a weight or water bottle in each hand with backs of hands facing forward and resting on thighs Ⓐ. Now breathe in and, as you breathe out, lift arms in front to shoulder height, keeping shoulders down, head up and elbows slightly bent Ⓑ. Lower again slowly and do 12 reps altogether. Rest before doing another 2 sets.

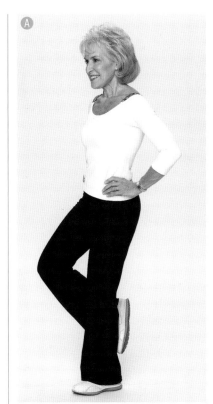

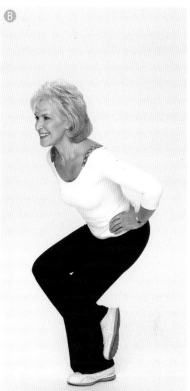

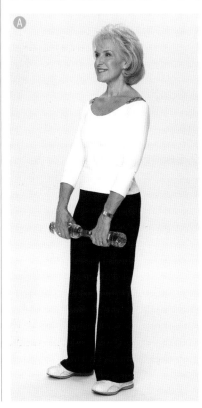

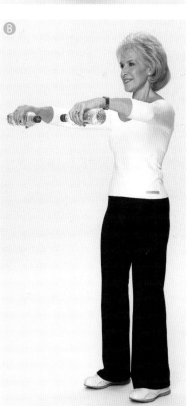

3 Spine stabiliser ▶

(× 10 reps alternate sides)
Come onto hands and knees with knees under hips and your shoulders over your wrists. Now slide right hand and left foot along the floor until leg and arm are as straight as possible Ⓐ. Hold tummy in tight, then lift leg and arm off floor in line with the trunk Ⓑ. Hold for 3 seconds, then release, and repeat on other side. Do 10 reps, changing sides each time.

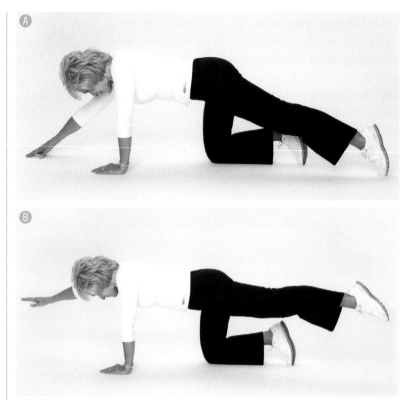

4 Bottom toner ▶

(× 12 reps each leg)
Start on forearms and knees, with knees under hips and your shoulders over your elbows, and extend left foot along floor Ⓐ. Pulling tummy in tight and keeping hips facing floor, lift leg in line with hip, leading with the heel Ⓑ. Lower again under control and continue lifting and lowering for 12 reps. Change legs and repeat.

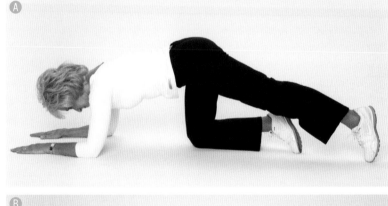

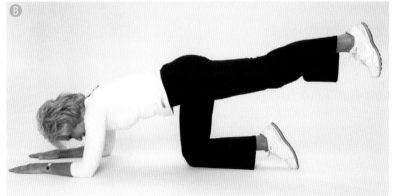

5 Tummy flattener

(× 4 reps)

Lie on front and lift onto forearms and knees, with toes curled under. Now breathe in and, as you breathe out, pull tummy in very tight and lift knees off floor so your body forms a straight line from top of head to feet. Hold for 10 seconds, then release. Do 4 reps.

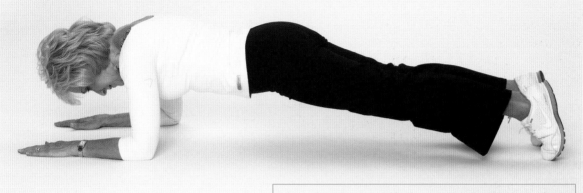

If you find this too difficult, keep your knees on the floor.

POST-WORKOUT STRETCHES

1 Front thigh stretch ▶

Lie on front, bend one knee and take hold of foot with hand on same side (or hold on to trouser leg or sock). Relax your upper body and gently press hip into floor to feel a stretch down front of thigh. Hold for 10 seconds, then change legs and repeat.

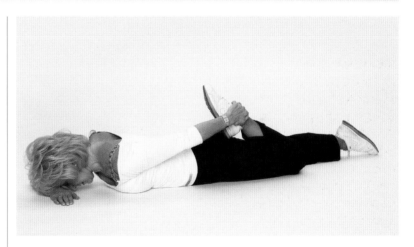

2 Tummy stretch ▶

Lie on your front with arms bent at sides. Now prop yourself up on elbows, keeping hips in contact with floor, and lift chin forward slightly to feel a stretch in your tummy. Hold for 10 seconds, then release.

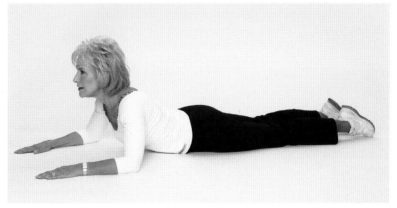

3 Back stretch ▶

Come up onto your hands and knees and, as you pull your tummy in, arch your spine up towards the ceiling, letting your head drop down. Hold for 10 seconds, then release.

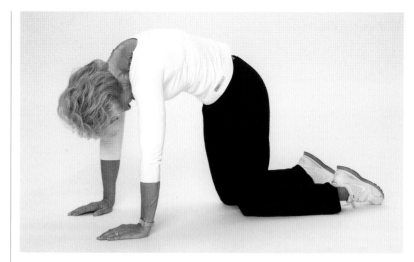

4 Back thigh stretch ▶

Sit upright with one leg straight out in front and the other bent. Place hands on floor at either side of straight leg and lean forward from hips to feel a stretch in back of thigh. Hold for 10 seconds, then try to lean a little further forward for another 10 seconds. Change legs and repeat.

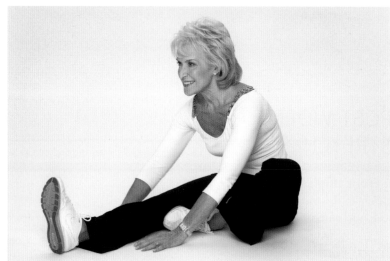

5 Chest stretch ▶

Sit upright and place both hands behind you on floor. Draw shoulders back to feel a stretch across chest, and hold for 10 seconds.

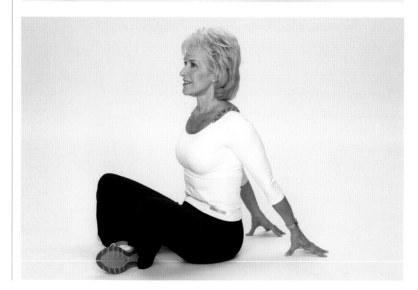

AEROBIC CHALLENGE

Go swimming, cycling, jogging, or anything that causes you to become mildly breathless. Try and work out for 30 minutes and remember to do your stretches at the end (see pp.177–9).

Exercise tip

Research has shown that couples are more likely to enjoy greater success on a first date if they do something active, e.g. a game of sport, walking or dancing, rather than having a passive evening watching a film or dining out. The physical activity acts as an alternative focal point and we can learn a lot about the other person when interacting in this way.

MOTIVATIONAL THOUGHT FOR THE DAY

We often say we don't have time to exercise, yet in the UK we watch an average of three hours of television a day!

I believe the main reason we don't exercise as much as we should is that many of us don't find a form of exercise that we really enjoy. We can buy the latest hi-tech exercise bike/treadmill/rowing machine, but after the first flurry of activity, it tends to be demoted to the garage, loft, spare bedroom or used as a clothes horse. Why? Because many people find them deadly boring! Men are much more likely to increase their fitness by playing a sport such as tennis, golf, badminton or squash – sports that are competitive, fun and also great workouts. Some people love swimming and can swim up to 40 lengths at a time. And the reason many people enjoy working out to a fitness DVD or attending an aerobics class is that they have to use their brains as well as their bodies to coordinate the moves. This is both stimulating and interesting and means they don't get bored.

During this four-week programme I have given you a specific exercise challenge each day and, because each day's challenge is different and gets more demanding as you progress, it becomes interesting as well as, hopefully, rewarding. At the end of this week you will need to decide what activity you are going to do on an ongoing basis.

Attending a Rosemary Conley Diet and Fitness Club class is one of the best things you could do as you will be personally supervised to ensure you do the exercises correctly. The workout at these classes, and in any of my DVDs, uses all the muscles in the body and provides an efficient all-round fitness training activity that incorporates fat burning and body toning exercises as well as a stretch session to increase flexibility. Add some regular brisk walking and perhaps an active sport or hobby, and you will be doing sufficient activity to help you continue to lose weight and maintain your new weight and your figure long term.

Day 26

Just three days to go – three crucial days until the end of this 28-day marathon! If you are still with me, I am so proud of you and you will be thrilled with the end results. However, you will need to be prepared for temptation to come knocking at your door at some point in the future to tease you away from your successful challenge. So put on your metaphorical bullet-proof vest and the arrows of temptation will just bounce off you and you will stay focused.

Plan to have a celebratory meal on Day 29 and treat yourself to some champagne. You will thoroughly deserve it. But for now, stick to the diet and be as active as you can. There are no toning exercises today, so give today's aerobic challenge your best effort. Enjoy your day!

MENU

Breakfast
■ 2 low-fat (max. 5 % fat) beef, pork or Quorn sausages, grilled, served with 1 yellow Portion Pot® (115g) baked beans and 50g grilled mushrooms ☑ P

Mid-morning power snack
■ 1 red Portion Pot® (115g) raspberries topped with 2 tsps low-fat yogurt (max. 5 % fat) ☑

Lunch
■ 2-egg omelette made using milk from allowance and lots of freshly ground black pepper, and filled with chopped peppers, red onion, mushrooms and 25g grated low-fat cheese (max. 5 % fat) ☑ P

Mid-afternoon power snack
■ 1 Hartley's Low Calorie Jelly topped with 1 tbsp Total 2 % Greek Yoghurt and 3 berries of your choice

Dinner
■ 175g lean beef fillet or rump steak or 2 Quorn Peppered Steaks, grilled, served with a large salad plus 1 tbsp Hellmann's Extra Light Mayonnaise ☑ P
OR
■ Cauliflower Bhaji (see recipe, p.221) served with 1 blue Portion Pot® (55g uncooked weight) or 1 red Portion Pot® (144g cooked weight) basmati rice per person ☑

Dessert
■ 1 × 120g pot Del Monte Fruitini Fruit Pieces in juice ☑

Alcohol or high-fat treat
■ 1 yellow Portion Pot® (125ml) red or white wine
OR
■ 1 × 21g bag Boots Shapers Salt & Vinegar Chipsticks ☑

WARM-UP

March on spot with shoulder rolls

Stand tall and march on the spot for a total of 2 minutes. For every 4 steps, do a full shoulder roll, pulling shoulders forward, up, back and down.

AEROBIC DAY

Choose any physical activity you like that is going to make you slightly breathless but that you can sustain for 45 minutes.

POST-AEROBIC STRETCHES

1 Calf stretch ▶

Place one foot in front of the other, with both feet pointing forward (hold on to a wall or sturdy surface for support if you wish). Bend front knee in line with ankle and keep back leg straight with heel pressing down. Lean further forward to feel a stretch in calf of back leg and hold for 10 seconds. Do the lower calf stretch before changing legs.

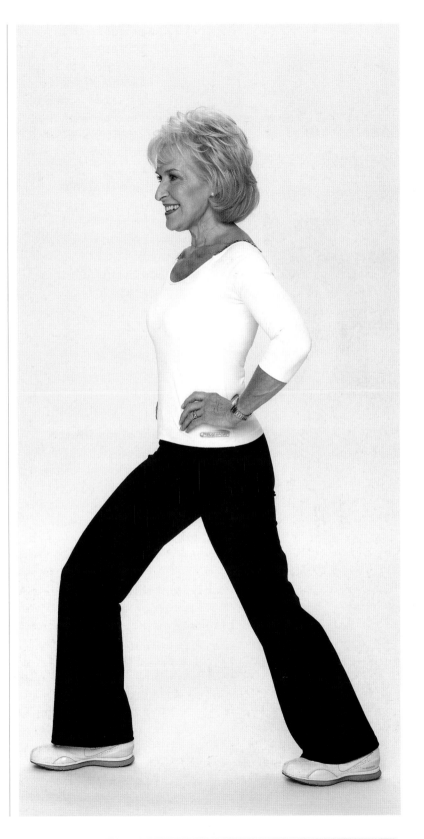

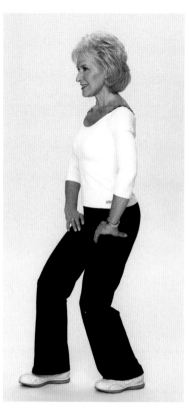

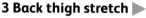 **2 Lower calf stretch**

Bring your back foot half a step in and bend both knees with feet still pointing forward. Keep both heels on floor and your body upright as you look straight ahead and hold for 10 seconds. Change legs and repeat both calf stretches.

3 Back thigh stretch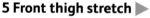

Straighten your front leg and keep your back leg bent. With spine straight, lean forward slightly to feel a stretch in back thigh of straight leg. Hold for 10 seconds, then change legs and repeat.

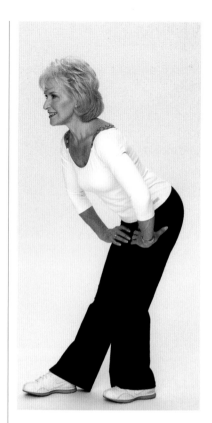

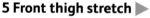 **4 Front of hip stretch**

Bend front leg and lift heel of back foot. With your weight equally distributed between both legs, trunk upright and tummy in, press pelvis forward to feel a stretch at top of hip. Hold for 10 seconds, then change legs and repeat.

5 Front thigh stretch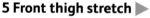

Stand upright and take hold of one ankle with hand (place other hand on wall or back of chair for support if necessary). Bring knees in line with each other and keep supporting leg slightly bent. Gently push hip of raised leg forward to stretch front of thigh. Hold stretch for 10 seconds, then change legs and repeat.

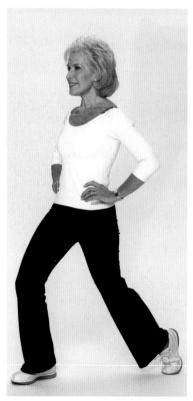

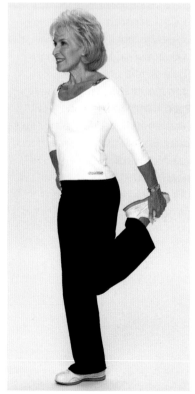

6 Inner thigh stretch ▶

Stand tall and take legs out wide. Bend one knee in line with ankle, keeping other leg straight with foot pointing forward, to feel a stretch in inner thigh of straight leg. Hold for 10 seconds, then change legs and repeat.

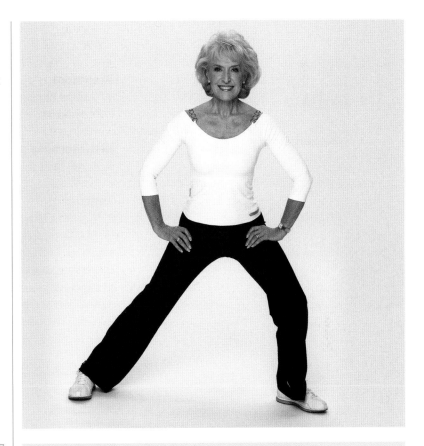

Exercise tip

Having the right shoes and fitness gear can increase our motivation to exercise. They don't need to be exotic, just comfortable and flattering. Now that you are slimmer, why not treat yourself?

MOTIVATIONAL THOUGHT FOR THE DAY

Over the last four weeks you will have dropped at least one dress size. Why not look for something new to wear on Day 29 that will show off your new, slimmer figure? Remember, if you have still a significant amount of excess weight to lose, have a look in a dress agency, where nearly-new clothes are sold at a fraction of the original cost, or in a charity shop where clothes can be had at bargain prices, to see if there is something that fits you for now and that you can recycle once you have lost more weight.

Plan to give yourself a mini-makeover on Day 29. Think about having your hair restyled, and perhaps having a professional make-up session – or at least treat yourself to some new products. If you make a real effort it will give you extra confidence and show the world that you are proud of what you have achieved over the last four weeks.

As these last few days creep up on you, it is good to keep your mind occupied with thoughts of these exciting treats rather than treats in the form of food!

Day 27

Only two days of the 28-day programme to go. For every day that you complete on this programme you are taking a very significant step towards your ultimate success because if you can give yourself the very best start to your weight-loss plan, you are much more likely to succeed in the long term. This four-week challenge – and no one is denying that it is challenging – provides you with a cracking start that will make a real difference to your health, your fitness and your size. So stay focused.

I have extended the toning session on these last couple of days to cover more muscle groups so that by the end of tomorrow you will have worked the whole body with these very advanced exercises. Give them your best effort and realise how much stronger your muscles are now compared to when you started the programme. Do not falter! Be as active as you can and continue planning your celebrations for Day 29.

MENU

Breakfast
- 1 yellow Portion Pot® (30g) All-Bran served with milk from allowance and 1 tsp sugar, plus 1 boiled egg ✓

Mid-morning power snack
- ½ grapefruit sprinkled with 1 tsp sugar ✓

Lunch
- Stir-Fried Chicken: Stir-fry 100g chopped chicken breast (no skin) in a preheated non-stick wok or pan without any added fat. Add some crushed garlic and, when the chicken has changed colour and is almost cooked through, add some chopped peppers, celery, red onion, mushrooms and mangetout, taking care not to overcook the veg. Just before serving, add some grated ginger, soy sauce and fresh coriander and heat through ℗
OR
- 1 slice wholegrain bread, toasted, topped with 1 × 300g can Heinz BBQ baked beans and 1 dry-fried small egg ✓

Mid-afternoon power snack
- 1 yellow Portion Pot® (125ml) apple juice ✓

Dinner
- 1 × 150g lean lamb steak (raw weight) or 2 Quorn Lamb Style Grills, grilled, served with 115g boiled new potatoes (with skins), plus 200g other vegetables of your choice and a little low-fat gravy and mint sauce ✓
OR
- Wine Braised Pork Slices (see recipe, p.215) served with 115g boiled new potatoes (with skins) and additional other vegetables of your choice

Dessert
- 1 The Skinny Cow Triple Chocolate Stick

Alcohol or high-fat treat
- 50ml measure of gin or vodka with a Slimline mixer
OR
- 1 × 25g bag Walkers Squares Cheese & Onion Flavour Potato Snack

WARM-UP

Knee lifts with pull-downs

Stand upright with hands above head and tummy pulled in. Lift alternate knees and as you lift each knee, pull your arms down to either side of the knees. Keep your tummy in and your back straight and continue for 1 minute.

FIVE-MINUTE TONE-UP – ADVANCED

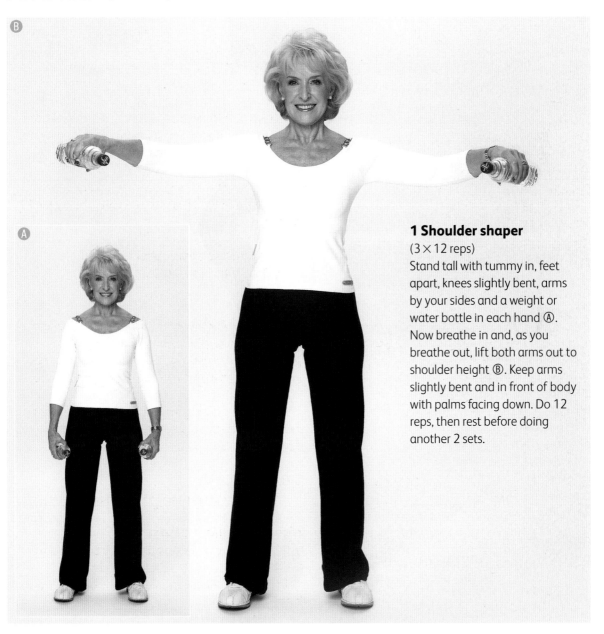

1 Shoulder shaper

(3 × 12 reps)

Stand tall with tummy in, feet apart, knees slightly bent, arms by your sides and a weight or water bottle in each hand Ⓐ. Now breathe in and, as you breathe out, lift both arms out to shoulder height Ⓑ. Keep arms slightly bent and in front of body with palms facing down. Do 12 reps, then rest before doing another 2 sets.

2 Tummy crunch ▶

(2 × 10 reps)

Lie on back with legs raised and ankles crossed. Place both hands behind head and pull tummy in tight Ⓐ. Now breathe out as you lift head and shoulders off floor and, at same time, lift hips slightly Ⓑ. Keep chin off chest and hold tummy in throughout. Do 10 reps, then rest before doing another set.

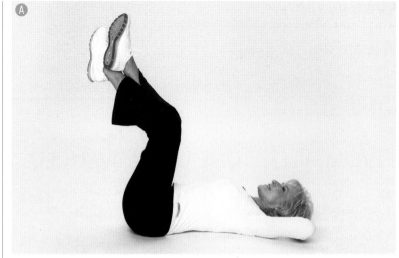

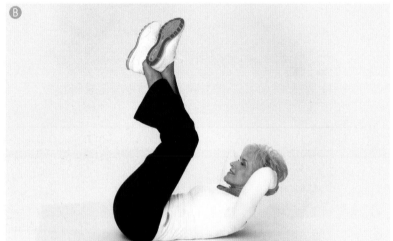

3 Advanced waist shaper ▶

(2 × 10 reps alternate sides)

Start in same position as Exercise 2. Breathe out and as you lift head and shoulders off floor, reach one arm up and across towards opposite foot. Lower again, then repeat to other side . Keep changing sides for 10 reps, then rest before doing another set.

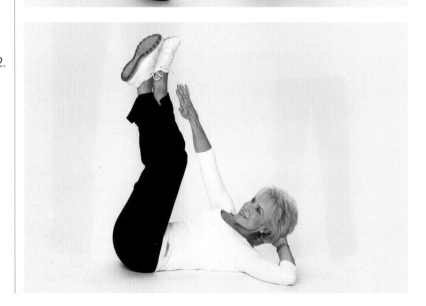

4 Outer thigh shaper ▶ with three-stage lift

(× 12 reps each leg)

Lie on side, bend bottom leg up to 90 degrees and push top leg out straight in line with hip, foot flexed, and hold a weight or water bottle on thigh. Pull tummy in to hold trunk still, then lift top leg slightly and pause Ⓐ. Now lift leg to mid range and pause Ⓑ, then lift to top of range and pause Ⓒ, keeping hips stacked. Lower under control in one movement, and repeat. Do 12 reps on one leg, then roll over and repeat on other leg.

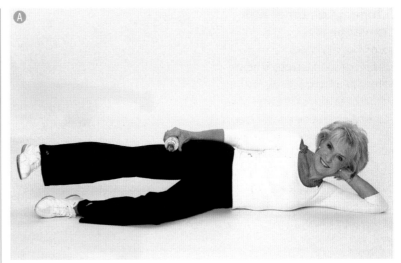

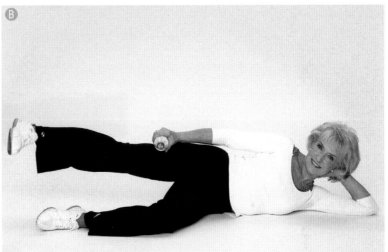

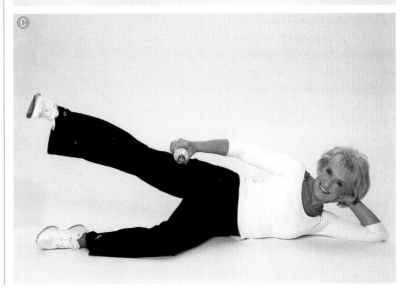

5 Inner thigh toner with ▶ two-stage lift

(× 16 reps each leg)

Lie on side propped up on elbow, with top leg bent over bottom leg and knee resting on a rolled towel. Straighten bottom leg and keep it off floor slightly Ⓐ. Pulling tummy in to keep trunk still, lift bottom leg halfway up and pause Ⓑ, then lift to top of range Ⓒ before lowering again with a pause halfway down. Do 16 reps, then roll over, change legs and repeat.

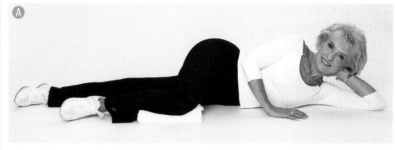

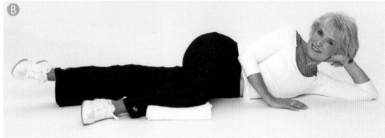

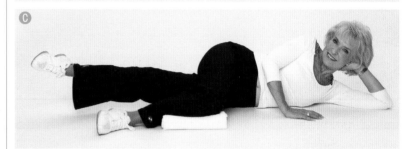

6 Full press-up ▶

(2 × 4 reps)

Come up onto hands and knees then straighten legs out behind, keeping body in line from head to feet Ⓐ. Now breathe in and bend elbows outward, lowering trunk to floor Ⓑ and holding tummy in to support your back. Breathe out as you push up again. Do 4 reps, then rest before doing another set.

If a full press-up is too difficult, repeat Exercise 5 (Chest and underarm toner) on Day 22, p.155.

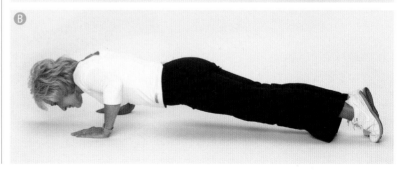

7 Posture improver and ▶ back strengthener

(3 × 6 reps)
Lie on front with arms by sides Ⓐ. Breathe out as you pull shoulders up and away from floor Ⓑ, then lift head off floor but keep looking down, with head in line with spine Ⓒ. Hold for 2 seconds, then breathe in and lower slowly. Do 6 reps, then rest before doing 2 more sets.

POST-WORKOUT STRETCHES

1 Tummy stretch ▼

Lie on front with arms at sides and elbows bent. Now prop up on your elbows, keeping hips in contact with floor, and lift your chin forward slightly to feel a stretch in your tummy. Hold for 10 seconds, then release.

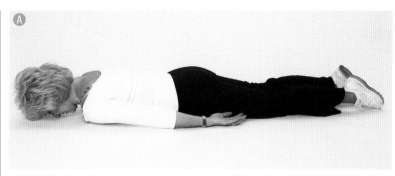

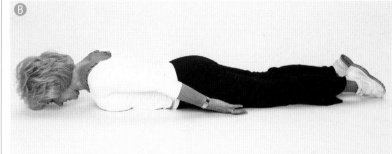

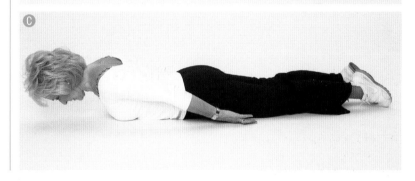

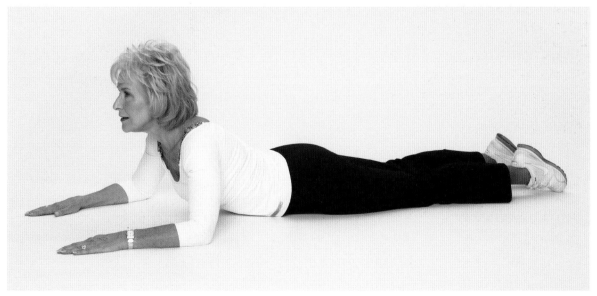

2 Back stretch ▶

Come up onto hands and knees and, as you pull your tummy in, arch your spine up towards the ceiling, letting your head drop down. Hold for 10 seconds, then release.

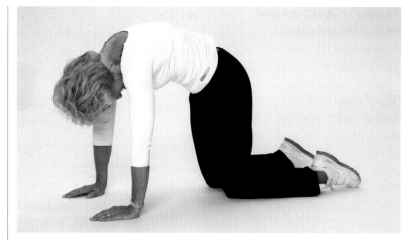

3 Waist stretch ▶

Still sitting up tall with legs crossed, lift right arm and lean over to left side, keeping both hips on floor and without leaning forward or back. Hold for 10 seconds, then change sides and repeat.

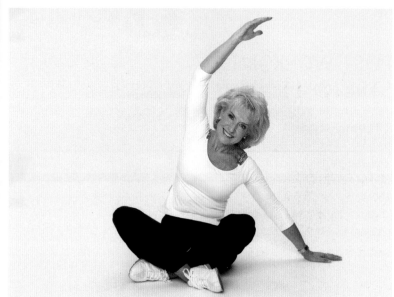

4 Chest stretch ▶

Still sitting upright with legs crossed, place both hands behind you on floor. Draw shoulders back to feel a stretch across the chest, and hold for 10 seconds.

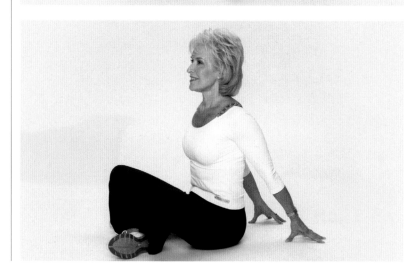

5 Underarm stretch ▼

Place right hand behind right shoulder and use pressure of left hand on right underarm to press right hand further down your back. Keep your head up and look straight ahead. Hold for 10 seconds, then change arms and repeat.

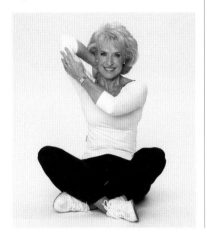

6 Inner thigh stretch

Sit with legs out wide and hands on floor behind hips. Now push hands into floor to help you sit upright, then lean forward from hips, keeping your back straight and head up, to stretch inner thighs. Hold stretch for 10 seconds, then breathe in and, as you breathe out, lean further forward for a stronger stretch and hold for another 10 seconds.

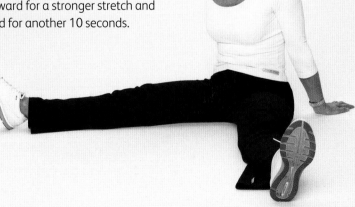

AEROBIC CHALLENGE

Do a 40-minute workout at a class or to a fitness DVD or go for a 30-minute brisk walk. Don't forget to stretch at the end.

Exercise tip

Plan to do tomorrow's exercises first thing in the morning, then they're done and you'll be less likely to sabotage your eating if you've risen early to work out.

MOTIVATIONAL THOUGHT FOR THE DAY

Today try on a garment that was a really tight fit on Day 1 and realise how many inches you have lost. It's very illuminating and satisfying to see the tangible difference in the fit of an item of clothing that was uncomfortably tight a month ago and that is very comfortably loose now.

Then pick up your 'weight-loss' bag in which you have placed the equivalent of your weight lost over the last three weeks and feel how heavy it is. Can you believe that you were once carrying that excess baggage around with you everywhere you went? No wonder you were tired and uncomfortable! In two days' time you will be adding even more weight to the bag and I hope you will be really impressed with your progress.

Try to work really hard today as every extra calorie you spend through activity will help minimise your body weight on the morning of Day 29 and maximise your results. Keep moving, keep smiling and look forward to your celebratory meal on Day 29.

Day 28

This is the last day of the 14-Day 1400 plan and perhaps the toughest bit of this eating plan. From tomorrow, though, if your personal calorie allowance permits, you will be able to eat more while continuing to lose weight. By the end of today you will have completed a very significant personal challenge and you can be proud of your efforts. Moreover you will have got your weight loss campaign off to a stunning start. Of course, you may not have much more weight to lose and you may even be happy with where you have now arrived, weight-wise. If so, please keep up the low-fat way of eating combined with regular activity so that it forms part of your everyday lifestyle.

Today's exercise plan runs through many of the toning exercises at their most challenging level and they will demonstrate how strong your muscles have become in just four weeks. Having strong muscles gives us a better shape and it makes weight loss and weight maintenance easier.

MENU

Breakfast
- Fruit Smoothie: Blend 150g peaches, strawberries, raspberries or blueberries with 100g Total 2% fat Greek Yoghurt and milk from allowance ☑

Mid-morning power snack
- 1 blue Portion Pot® (14g) Special K (eat dry or with milk from allowance) ☑

Lunch
- 1 × 400g can any lentil or bean soup (max. 350 kcal and 5% fat), plus 1 piece fresh fruit (excluding bananas) ☑

OR
- 1 pack Rosemary Conley Solo Slim Soup: choose from Tomato, Pea and Ham, Three Bean and Chorizo, Mushroom or Minestrone (order from www.rosemaryconley.com), plus 1 slice wholegrain bread and 1 piece fresh fruit

Mid-afternoon power snack
- 1 small bowl of mixed salad tossed in fat-free dressing ☑

Dinner
- Sweet and Sour Pork Chop: Grill 1 × 140g lean pork chop, all visible fat removed, and serve with 115g boiled new potatoes (with skins), 100g each carrots and broccoli, plus 1 yellow Portion Pot® (125ml) Uncle Ben's Sweet & Sour Light sauce

OR
- Barbecued Garlic Chicken (see recipe, p.212) served with 100g boiled new potatoes (with skins) plus salad or vegetables

Dessert
- 1 meringue basket filled with 1 tsp 0% fat Greek yogurt and topped with 1 slice pineapple ☑

Alcohol or high-fat treat
- 1 yellow Portion Pot® (125ml) glass champagne

OR
- 1 × 20g fun-size bag M & Ms

WARM-UP

Twisted canoeing

Stand tall and bring both arms overhead with tummy in. Now drop both arms to one side as you bend knees and hips, then come up and repeat, dropping arms to other side. Keep going for 1 minute.

FIVE-MINUTE TONE-UP – ADVANCED

1 Front shoulder shaper ▶

(3 × 12 reps)

Stand tall with back straight and hold a weight or water bottle in each hand with backs of hands facing forward and resting on front of thighs Ⓐ. Now breathe in and, as you breathe out, lift arms in front to shoulder height, keeping shoulders down, head up and elbows slightly bent Ⓑ. Lower again slowly and do 12 reps altogether. Rest before doing another 2 sets.

2 One-legged squat ▶

(2 × 6 reps each leg)

Stand tall with hands on hips or on back of a chair for support. Place right foot behind left ankle and pull tummy in to help you balance Ⓐ. Now bend left knee, pushing hips back Ⓑ. Come up again without locking knee of supporting leg. Do 6 reps slowly, then change legs and repeat. Rest before doing another set.

> If balancing on one leg is too difficult, keep both feet on floor.

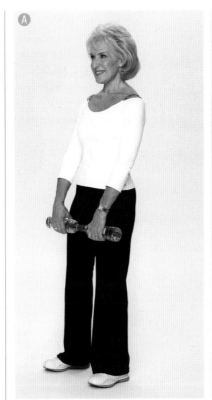
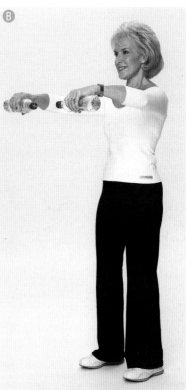
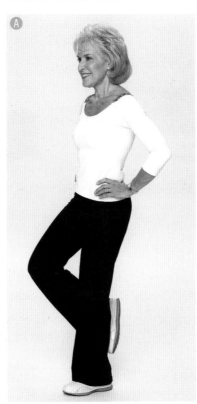
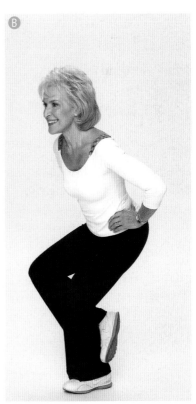

3 Waist cycling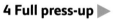

(2 × 12 reps alternate sides)
Lie on back with feet off floor and legs at 90 degrees. Place hands behind head and pull tummy in tight Ⓐ. Breathe in and, as you breathe out, lift head and shoulders off floor and, at same time, bring right shoulder towards left knee and straighten right leg to form 45-degree angle with floor Ⓑ. Keep head and shoulders off floor as you repeat to other side. Continue to change sides, keeping hips on floor to prevent rolling from side to side. Do 12 reps (6 each side), then rest before doing another set.

> If cycling is too difficult, keep your legs stationary at 90 degrees and just raise shoulder towards opposite knee.

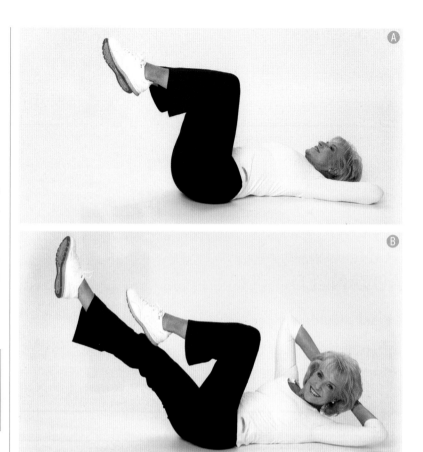

4 Full press-up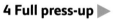

(3 × 4 reps)
Come up onto hands and knees then straighten legs out behind, keeping body in line from head to feet Ⓐ. Now breathe in and bend elbows outward, lowering trunk to floor Ⓑ and holding tummy in to support your back. Breathe out as you push up again. Do 4 reps, then rest before doing another 2 sets.

> If a full press-up is too difficult, repeat Exercise 5 (Chest and underarm toner) from Day 22, p.155.

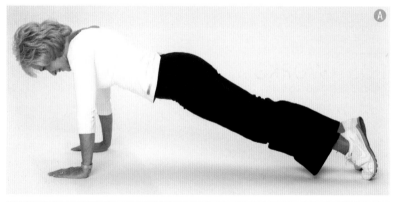

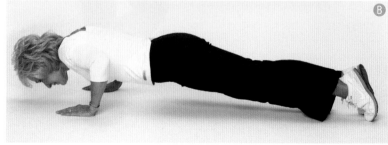

5 Bottom lifter ▶

(2 × 6 reps)

Lie on front with head resting on hands and both legs out straight and wide Ⓐ. Now, pulling tummy in and keeping upper body relaxed, push both legs away so they start to lift off floor no higher than length of foot Ⓑ. Hold for a second at the top, then lower your legs under control. Do 6 reps, then rest before doing another set.

> If lifting both legs together is too difficult, just lift one leg at a time.

6 Tummy flattener ▶

(× 4 reps)

Lie on front and lift onto forearms and knees, with toes curled under. Now breathe in and, as you breathe out, pull tummy in very tight and lift knees off floor so your body forms a straight line from top of head to feet. Hold for 10 seconds, then release. Do 4 reps.

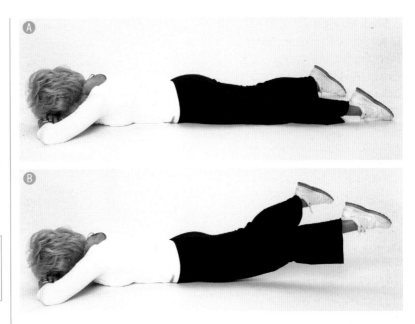

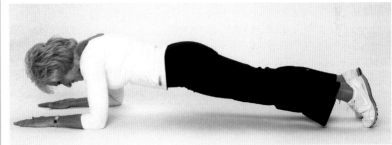

> If you find this exercise too difficult, keep your knees on the floor.

POST-WORKOUT STRETCHES

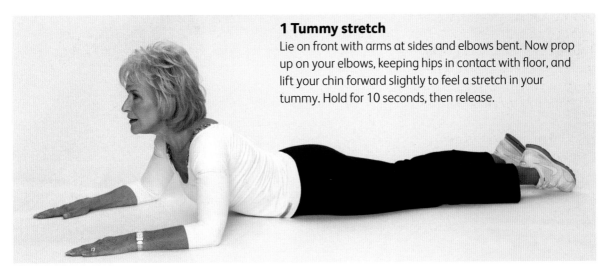

1 Tummy stretch

Lie on front with arms at sides and elbows bent. Now prop up on your elbows, keeping hips in contact with floor, and lift your chin forward slightly to feel a stretch in your tummy. Hold for 10 seconds, then release.

2 Back stretch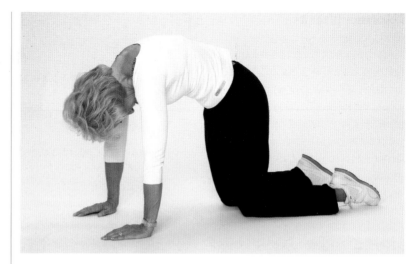

Come up onto your hands and knees and, as you pull your tummy in, arch your spine up towards the ceiling, letting your head drop down. Hold for 10 seconds, then release.

3 Front thigh stretch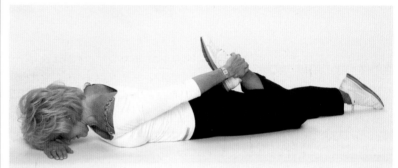

Lie on front, bend one knee and take hold of foot with hand on same side (or hold on to trouser leg or sock). Relax your upper body and gently press hip into floor to feel a stretch down front of thigh. Hold for 10 seconds, then change legs and repeat.

4 Waist stretch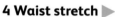

Still sitting up tall with legs crossed, lift right arm and lean over to left side, keeping both hips on floor and without leaning forward or back. Hold for 10 seconds, then change sides and repeat.

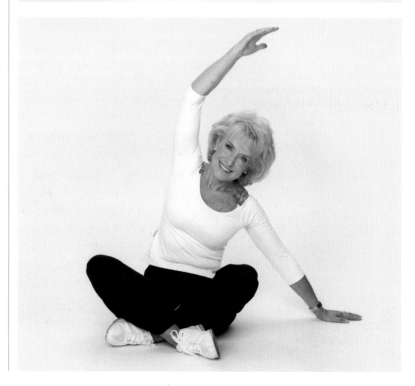

5 Underarm stretch ▼

Still sitting upright with legs crossed, place right hand behind right shoulder. Use pressure of left hand on right underarm to press right hand further down your back. Keep your head up and look straight ahead. Hold for 10 seconds, then change arms and repeat.

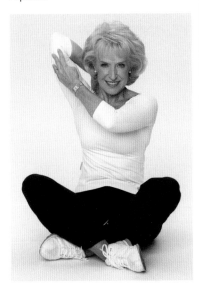

6 Chest stretch ▼

Sit upright and place both hands behind you on floor. Draw shoulders back to feel a stretch across chest, and hold for 10 seconds.

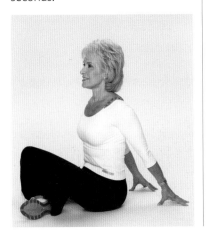

AEROBIC CHALLENGE

Walk up and down stairs 5 times consecutively, twice throughout the day, plus take a 30-minute brisk walk or jog. Really go for it!

> **Exercise tip**
> Taking regular exercise will help to lower your cholesterol and blood pressure levels as well as burn extra calories and tone your muscles, so the benefits of continuing to exercise even after you have achieved your goal weight are enormous.

MOTIVATIONAL THOUGHT FOR THE DAY

Over the last four weeks you will have burned a lot of body fat through eating healthily and doing aerobic exercise. Your heart and lungs will have become fitter and more efficient and your skin will be looking much clearer.

The toning exercises that you have done almost every day will have strengthened your muscles considerably and caused them to become tighter and more efficient. If muscles are not worked, they will become smaller through wastage – and that's the last thing you need when you are trying to lose weight.

We need strong muscles for several reasons. Our muscles help us to move about, bend, carry things and complete all manner of functions in our everyday lives and if we don't keep our muscles strong, we will become weaker and less mobile. As muscle is energy-hungry tissue, so strong muscles also give us a higher metabolic rate, which helps us to burn extra calories every day even when we are not exercising.

Remember also that muscles are our 'fat-burning machines'. When we do aerobic activity, the extra oxygen we breathe in enters our bloodstream via our arteries and flows around our body and into our muscles. Then the mitochondria ('little engines') in our muscles spring into action and, with the aid of the oxygen, burn body fat to make fuel for energy. So, be assured, exercise is the key to weight loss and weight maintenance.

Do as much aerobic activity today as you can. The scales and the tape measure will show the benefits to your figure tomorrow if you do.

Phase 3: Your personal inch loss plan

Congratulations! You've done it! Four weeks of serious dieting and a major exercise programme completed. Now life gets a little easier as you move on to this third phase. You must be delighted with what you have achieved – lots of inches have disappeared from your body and no doubt a considerable amount of weight too.

Day 29

In the morning, after you have visited the bathroom, head for those scales. The results at the end of the fourth week on a diet are unpredictable. People lose weight at different rates and of course much depends on how accurate you have been in measuring your food portions, how much exercise you have done and how much you weighed in the first place.

Whatever you have lost – whether a big drop or just a few pounds – it is a significant milestone and you should be delighted. I really hope you are.

Now measure yourself with your tape measure or Magic Measure® and take a good look at how many inches you have lost from the different areas of your body. Get out your measuring belt and see where it fits around your waist. Record your results on your chart or in your journal.

Next, find something of equivalent weight to this week's loss to place in your 'weight-loss' bag, then lift it up. Savour the moment as you realise the superb results of your hard work and determination.

If possible, at some point today, take a photograph of yourself or get someone else to do it. Compare it with your original 'before' photograph that you took before you started the diet. The difference you can see should be very encouraging. From now on, take a photograph every month as you continue on the diet.

Working out your calorie allowance

To calculate your new personalised calorie allowance, turn to page 230. Look at the column appropriate to your gender and age and then find your today's weight, or the nearest weight to it, on the table. This figure is your BMR (basal metabolic rate) calculation, which is the number of calories your body would burn if you stayed in bed all day and did nothing.

By eating this number of calories you will be meeting your basic metabolic needs and the bulk of those calories need to be taken in the form of proper, nutritious food – rather than alcohol, high-fat snacks or sugar. Your body will effectively then draw down your body fat to burn as extra fuel to make up the shortfall of calories you will be spending as you move about during the day and hopefully doing some exercise too.

As you lose each further half stone, you should adjust your calories accordingly. Sorry – but the slimmer you become, the fewer calories you have to eat if you want to keep losing weight at the same rate. An alternative would be to keep increasing your calorie output by doing extra exercise on top of what you are already doing.

Continue to exercise regularly. You can repeat the last two weeks of the 28-day exercise programme if you wish. Alternatively, you can choose any other activity you enjoy. As long as you combine some aerobic work with toning and strength exercises you will keep progressing and enjoying the benefits.

How to design your own plan

You can select any breakfast, lunch and dinner from the suggestions on the following pages. You will find more calorie-counted recipes on www.rosemaryconley.com and on our online TV channel www.rosemaryconley.tv where chef Dean Simpole-Clarke demonstrates how to prepare all the recipes in this book plus hundreds of additional low-fat recipes that will fit in with this diet.

For a diet to work it must offer foods that you enjoy. As long as the calories are counted and the fat content of each meal is five per cent or less (5 grams of fat per 100 grams of product), you cannot go wrong. This diet has to be the most versatile ever. If there's a meal you don't like, you don't have to eat it, ever!

Always drink plenty of water and be sure to consume 450ml (¾ pint) skimmed or semi-skimmed milk every day to ensure you get sufficient calcium. Keep taking a multivitamin supplement just to be super-sure that you have all the necessary micronutrients for good health. If you eat similar foods all the time, because you like them, you could be missing out on some important vitamins and minerals.

If you have extra calories available, over and above the 1200 calories used within the basic diet, you can use these for an alcoholic drink, a low-fat dessert or treat and, remember, you can use 100 calories a day for a high-fat treat of your choice.

Don't exceed your daily calorie allowance unless you have saved up any calories during the week. It can be useful to have calories available for a party or special night out with friends, but if you abuse your treats allowance you will stop losing weight and you may find yourself falling back into old, high-fat, habits. It's just not worth it.

Diet menus

BREAKFASTS

Cereal breakfasts

■ 1 green Portion Pot® (50g) Special K cereal plus milk from allowance and 1 tsp sugar ☑

■ 1 yellow Portion Pot® (30g) fruit and fibre cereal served with milk from allowance and topped with 1 red Portion Pot® (115g) fresh raspberries or 1 tsp sugar ☑

■ 1 red Portion Pot® (50g) fruit and fibre cereal (or any bran cereal), served with milk from allowance and 10 seedless grapes ☑

■ 1 Weetabix or Shredded Wheat served with milk from allowance plus 1 tsp sugar and 1 thinly sliced medium banana ☑

■ 2 Weetabix served with milk from allowance and 2 tsps sugar or 1 mini banana ☑

■ 1 yellow Portion Pot® (14 Minis) Weetabix Fruit 'n' Nut Minis, plus 1 medium banana, sliced, served with milk from allowance ☑

■ 1 yellow Portion Pot® (30g) All-Bran served with milk from allowance and 1 tsp sugar, plus 1 boiled egg ☑

■ 1 red Portion Pot® (30g) Sugar Puffs mixed with 115g canned peaches in natural juice ☑

■ Mix 100g 0% fat Greek yogurt with 1 blue Portion Pot® (40g) muesli and a little semi-skimmed milk from allowance to moisten. Add a little Silver Spoon Half Spoon to sweeten to taste. Leave to soak overnight in the refrigerator for best results. Serve chilled ☑

■ 1 blue Portion Pot® (35g) uncooked porridge oats, cooked in water with 10 sultanas and served with milk from allowance ☑

Fruit breakfasts

■ 1 Müllerlight yogurt, any flavour (max. 150 kcal), plus 1 small banana

■ 2 large bananas ☑

■ Frozen Berry Smoothie (see recipe, p.225) ☑

■ Fruit Smoothie: blend 150g fresh fruit (peaches, strawberries, raspberries or blueberries) with 100g Total 2% fat Greek Yoghurt and milk from allowance ☑

■ 1 small banana, sliced, mixed with 115g sliced strawberries and 1 × 100g pot low-fat yogurt, any flavour (max. 100 kcal and 5% fat) ☑

■ 200g fresh fruit salad topped with 100g Total 2% fat Greek Yoghurt and 6 sultanas ☑

■ 100g Total 2% fat Greek Yoghurt mixed with 140g fresh fruit, sweetened to taste with a little Silver Spoon Half Spoon ☑

Quick and easy breakfasts

■ 1 yellow Portion Pot® (125ml) fresh orange juice, plus 1 slice wholegrain bread spread with 2 tsps marmalade, jam or honey ☑

■ ½ fresh grapefruit plus 2 boiled medium-sized eggs ☑ P

■ ½ bagel (or 1 whole mini bagel) toasted, spread with 1 tsp fruit preserve, jam, honey or marmalade, then topped with 50g Total 2% Greek Yoghurt ☑

■ 200g Total 2% fat Greek Yoghurt mixed with 1 tsp runny honey ☑

■ 4 prunes, soaked overnight in 1 blue Portion Pot® (80g) low-fat natural yogurt, mixed with 1 tsp porridge oats ☑

Cooked breakfasts

■ 2 well-grilled back bacon rashers or 2 Quorn sausages, grilled, served with 1 dry-fried medium-sized egg, 3 tomatoes, halved and grilled, and 5 grilled mushrooms ☑ P

■ 2 low-fat (max. 5% fat) beef, pork or Quorn sausages, grilled, served with 1 yellow Portion Pot® (115g) baked beans and 50g grilled mushrooms ☑ P

■ 2 Quorn sausages, grilled, served with 1 dry-fried medium-sized egg and 1 × 200g can tomatoes, boiled until reduced ☑ P

- 2 Quorn sausages, grilled, served with 1 × 400g can tomatoes boiled until reduced, plus 50g grilled mushrooms ☑ P
- 1 Quorn Bacon Style Rasher, grilled, served with 1 yellow Portion Pot® (115g) baked beans plus 1 tomato, halved and grilled, and 50g grilled mushrooms ☑ P
- Tomatoes and Mushrooms on Toast: Boil 1 × 400g can chopped tomatoes well to reduce to a thick consistency and season well with freshly ground black pepper. Spoon onto 1 toasted large slice wholegrain bread and serve with 10 grilled mushrooms ☑
- ½ fresh grapefruit plus 1 poached medium-sized egg served on 1 toasted small slice wholegrain bread spread with Marmite ☑
- 2 eggs scrambled with milk from allowance and served with 100g grilled tomatoes and unlimited grilled mushrooms ☑ P
- 2-egg omelette made using milk from allowance, dry-fried and filled with chopped mushrooms, sliced cherry tomatoes and freshly ground black pepper ☑
- 2 turkey rashers and 1 low-fat beef or pork sausage (max. 5% fat), grilled or dry-fried, served with 1 × 200g can tomatoes boiled until reduced and 100g grilled mushrooms P
- 4 turkey rashers, grilled, served with 100g grilled, sliced mushrooms and 2 large tomatoes, grilled ☑ P
- 4 turkey rashers, grilled, served with 1 dry-fried medium-sized egg, 1 × 200g can plum tomatoes, boiled until reduced, and 5 grilled mushrooms P
- 2 turkey rashers, grilled, served with 1 yellow Portion Pot® (115g) baked beans and 1 dry-fried medium-sized egg P
- 1 slice wholegrain bread, toasted, topped with 1 yellow Portion Pot® (115g) baked beans ☑
- 1 slice wholegrain bread, soaked in 1 beaten egg and milk from allowance, fried in a little spray oil and topped with 1 tsp maple syrup ☑
- 1 small slice multigrain bread, toasted, served with 1 egg, scrambled, boiled or dry-fried; plus ½ pink grapefruit ☑
- 1 slice wholegrain bread, toasted, spread with savoury sauce (e.g. tomato ketchup, brown sauce or fruity sauce), then topped with 2 grilled turkey rashers plus 3 grilled tomatoes
- 1 slice wholegrain bread, toasted, topped with 1 scrambled egg and 2 grilled tomatoes ☑
- 1 blue Portion Pot® (35g) uncooked porridge oats, cooked in water with 10 sultanas and served with milk from allowance ☑

LUNCHES

Sandwich lunches

■ Any pre-packed sandwich of your choice (max. 300 kcal and 5% fat) ☑

■ Spread 2 slices wholegrain bread with horseradish sauce or Hellmann's Extra Light Mayonnaise and make into a jumbo sandwich with 30g wafer thin beef, chicken or ham and salad vegetables

■ Cheese and Marmite Sandwich: Spread 2 slices wholegrain bread with Marmite and fill with 40g low-fat cottage cheese ☑

■ BLT Sandwich: Toast 2 slices wholegrain bread, then spread 1 slice with 1 tsp Hellmann's Extra Light Mayonnaise and the other with tomato ketchup and fill with 25g lean grilled bacon, 1 slice wafer thin chicken, lettuce leaves and sliced tomatoes

■ Spread 2 slices wholegrain bread with HP Fruity Sauce (or similar) and make into a sandwich with 3 grilled turkey rashers, then toast in a sandwich toaster or double-sided electric grill

■ 1 medium slice wholegrain bread, toasted, topped with 1 × 125g can sardines or mackerel fillets, plus a small salad

Rolls, bagels and baguettes

■ 1 small wholegrain roll spread with 1 tsp horseradish sauce and topped with 50g wafer thin beef and sliced tomatoes, plus a small salad tossed in fat-free dressing

■ 1 bagel cut in half, spread with 50g Philadelphia Extra Light soft cheese then topped with 50g smoked salmon and freshly ground black pepper or chopped fresh dill

■ 1 small granary baguette spread with 1 tsp horseradish sauce mixed with a little low-fat Greek yogurt and filled with 100g diced cooked beetroot, 50g smoked trout fillets plus rocket leaves and watercress

■ 1 × 40g granary baguette spread with 20g Philadelphia Extra Light soft cheese then topped with 25g wafer thin ham or Quorn Deli Ham Style, 1 sliced tomato and mustard to taste, plus a small side salad ☑

■ BLT Bruschetta: Cut 1 × 30g granary or wholegrain baguette in half and toast lightly, then spread with 2 tsps Hellmann's Extra Light Mayonnaise. Top with lettuce, sliced tomato and 2 × 15g extra lean grilled back bacon rashers

Pitta bread and wraps

■ 1 × 50g wholemeal pitta bread filled with 50g low-fat houmous and chopped mixed salad sprinkled with low-fat dressing of your choice ☑

■ 1 pitta bread, split open, then spread with low-fat Marie Rose dressing or very low-fat mayonnaise and filled with shredded lettuce, cherry tomatoes and 100g cooked prawns

■ Brunch Pitta (see recipe, p.216)

■ Prawn Wrap: Spread 1 tortilla wrap with 1 tsp Thai sweet chilli dipping sauce, then fill with 50g cooked prawns, chopped salad leaves, peppers, cucumber, celery and cherry tomatoes and wrap into a parcel before cutting in half horizontally to make 2 wraps

■ 1 tortilla wrap spread with 1 tsp Thai sweet chilli dipping sauce, then filled with 50g cooked prawns, chopped salad leaves, peppers, cucumber, celery and cherry tomatoes and wrapped into a parcel before cutting in half horizontally to make 2 wraps

■ Greek Salad Wrap (see recipe, p.222) ☑

Salad lunches

■ 100g cooked chicken breast (no skin), sliced, served with a large mixed salad and 1 tbsp Hellmann's Extra Light Mayonnaise 🅿

■ Large salad of grated carrots, beansprouts, chopped peppers, celery, tomatoes, cucumber and red onion, served with 1 blue Portion Pot® (100g) low-fat cottage cheese, plus 1 tbsp Hellmann's Extra Light Mayonnaise. Plus 1 low-fat yogurt (max. 100 kcal and 5% fat) ☑

■ Salad Bowl with Prawns, Chicken or Ham: Place a large selection of shredded salad leaves and fresh herbs such as coriander and basil in a serving dish. Add layers of chopped peppers, onion, celery, mushrooms, cucumber and cherry tomatoes and top with chopped fresh fruits such as pineapple, papaya, mango, kiwi. Add 50g cooked prawns or chicken or shredded ham, then pour some low-fat Marie Rose sauce or other low-fat dressing over the salad and sprinkle with chopped chives 🅿

■ Mixed Bean Salad: Mix together 100g drained, canned chickpeas, 100g red kidney beans and 25g sweetcorn kernels. Add 2 sliced spring onions, 3 halved cherry tomatoes, unlimited chopped celery, peppers and cucumber, and mix well. Stir in some chopped fresh coriander and basil and toss in balsamic vinegar or fat-free dressing of your choice and add freshly ground black pepper to taste ☑

■ 2 hard-boiled eggs served with salad of chopped vegetables and salad leaves, tossed in low-fat dressing of your choice. Plus 1 kiwi fruit and 1 small pear ☑ P

■ Large mixed salad plus 1 smoked mackerel fillet or 1 × 125g can sardines or salmon (not in oil), served with 2 tsps Hellmann's Extra Light Mayonnaise or other low-fat dressing of your choice. Plus 1 pear or orange P

■ 100g cooked prawns served with a large mixed salad and 1 tbsp low-fat thousand island dressing. Plus 1 Danone Shape Lasting Satisfaction or Weight Watchers yogurt, any flavour

Quick and easy lunches

■ 1 egg, scrambled, then mixed with 25g Rosemary Conley low-fat Mature Cheese and served on 1 toasted small slice multigrain bread with 1 sliced tomato

■ ½ × 410g can Stagg Vegetable Garden Vegetable Chilli and 1 small wholegrain roll plus a small salad tossed in fat-free dressing ☑

■ 1 slice wholegrain bread, toasted, topped with 1 × 300g can Heinz BBQ baked beans and 1 dry-fried small egg ☑

■ 1 yellow Portion Pot® (115g) baked beans served on 2 toasted slices multigrain bread ☑

■ 200g Total 2% fat Greek Yoghurt mixed with 1 tsp runny honey and 1 red Portion Pot® (115g) raspberries or chopped strawberries or 1 yellow Portion Pot® (70g) blueberries, topped with 1 tsp muesli ☑

Cooked lunches

■ 1 × 140g tuna steak, grilled, served with 100g cooked peas and 50g sweetcorn plus a small salad. Plus 100g Total 2% fat Greek Yoghurt mixed with 1 red Portion Pot® (115g) raspberries

■ 2-egg omelette made using milk from allowance and lots of freshly ground black pepper, filled with chopped peppers, red onion, mushrooms and 25g grated low-fat cheese (max. 5% fat, e.g. Rosemary Conley low-fat Mature Cheese) ☑ P

■ Spanish omelette: In a non-stick frying pan or omelette pan, cook 2 beaten eggs with chopped peppers and red onion and 1 sliced, small cooked new potato. Serve with a small mixed salad tossed in fat-free dressing ☑

■ 2 well-grilled back bacon rashers, grilled, served with 1 dry-fried medium-sized egg, 1 × 400g can plum tomatoes boiled and reduced and 100g grilled or boiled mushrooms

■ Chicken or Quorn Stir-Fry: Dry-fry 100g sliced chicken breast (no skin) or Quorn fillets in a non-stick pan, then add a selection of chopped vegetables (e.g. peppers, onions, carrots, courgettes, celery, beansprouts), plus soy sauce to taste and 2 tsps sweet chilli sauce, taking care not to overcook the vegetables. Plus 1 low-fat yogurt (max. 100 kcal and 5% fat) ☑ P

■ Turkey and Mango Samosas (see recipe, p.213) served with unlimited fresh vegetables or salad

■ Gammon and Liver Kebabs: Cut 1 × 100g gammon steak (all visible fat removed) and 125g lamb's liver into bite-sized pieces and thread alternately on to wooden skewers. Cook under a hot conventional grill for 3–4 minutes each side or in a health grill for 2 minutes. Serve with grilled tomatoes and mixed salad leaves P

■ Stir-Fried Chicken: Stir-fry 100g chopped chicken breast (no skin) in a preheated non-stick wok or pan without any added fat. Add some crushed garlic and, when the chicken has changed colour and is almost cooked through, add some chopped peppers, celery, red onion, mushrooms and mangetout, taking care not to overcook the vegetables. Just before serving, add some grated ginger, soy sauce and fresh coriander and heat through P

■ 2 low-fat beef or pork sausages (max. 5% fat) or 2 Quorn sausages, grilled, served with 1 yellow Portion Pot® (115g) baked beans, 1 dry-fried small egg, 1 small can tomatoes boiled well to reduce, plus unlimited grilled or boiled mushrooms ☑ P

- 1 × 175g oven-baked sweet potato topped with either 75g tuna or low-fat cottage cheese, mixed with 1 tbsp sweetcorn and 1 tbsp Hellmann's Extra Light Mayonnaise, served with a small salad tossed in fat-free dressing of your choice ☑
- 1 × 175g oven-baked sweet potato topped with 75g baked beans, served with a side salad tossed in fat-free dressing of your choice ☑

Pasta, rice and noodle lunches

- Chicken Pasta: Cook 1 yellow Portion Pot® (45g dry weight) pasta shapes, then mix with 50g cooked, chopped chicken breast (no skin). Add some chopped salad vegetables (onions, peppers, cucumber, tomatoes), mix in 4 tbsps Hellmann's Extra Light Mayonnaise and serve with a small mixed salad
- Pasta with Tomato and Basil Sauce: Boil 1 yellow Portion Pot® (45g uncooked weight) pasta shapes in water with a vegetable stock cube, then drain and mix with ½ × 340g jar (170g) tomato and basil pasta sauce ☑
- Tuna or Chicken Pasta Salad: 1 red Portion Pot® (110g cooked weight) pasta shapes mixed with either 50g drained canned tuna (in brine) or 30g chopped cooked chicken breast, plus unlimited chopped peppers, red onion, cucumber, tomato and celery and 2 tsps Hellmann's Extra Light Mayonnaise or low-fat thousand island dressing
- Smoked Salmon Pasta Salad: Toss 1 yellow Portion Pot® (45g uncooked weight) or 1 red Portion Pot® (110g cooked weight) boiled pasta shapes with 50g smoked salmon strips and 1 yellow Portion Pot® (135g) low-fat fromage frais and chopped fresh dill, and serve with a green salad
- Garlic Mushroom Pasta (see recipe, p.219) ☑
- Singapore Noodles with Prawns (see recipe, p.218) plus a crisp salad ☑
- Stir-Fried Rice Noodles (see recipe, p.221) served with salad ☑
- 75g cooked egg noodles tossed with unlimited beansprouts, spring onions, chopped peppers, fresh coriander and 75g flaked cooked salmon, served with soy sauce
- Chicken and Rice Salad: 80g (cooked weight) boiled basmati rice mixed with 60g cooked chopped chicken breast (no skin), chopped peppers, red onion,

mushrooms, celery and 1 tbsp sweetcorn kernels. Season with freshly ground black pepper and soy sauce or fat-free dressing of your choice
- Bombay Rice (see recipe, p.220) served with salad ☑

Soup lunches

- 1 × 400g can any soup (max. 150 kcal and 5% fat). Plus 1 Müllerlight yogurt, any flavour (max. 150 kcal)
- 1 can any lentil or bean soup (max. 300 kcal and 5% fat); followed by 2 pieces fresh fruit (excluding bananas) ☑
- 1 × 400g can any soup (max. 150 kcal and 5% fat). Plus 1 Müllerlight yogurt, any flavour (max. 150 kcal)
- 1 Batchelors Cup a Soup. Plus 1 Müllerlight yogurt (max. 150 kcal) and 1 kiwi fruit
- Homemade Vegetable Soup (makes enough for approx. 6 servings): Bring 2 litres of water to the boil in a large pan, then add 2 vegetable stock cubes and 400g peeled and trimmed vegetables (e.g. carrots, parsnips, onion, cabbage) or leftover vegetables and boil until cooked. Remove from the heat, add some chopped coriander and black pepper and leave to cool a little. Pour the soup in small batches in a food processor and blend for a few seconds, then transfer to a storage container or jug and allow to cool before storing or freezing. Reheat as required, allowing 300ml per serving and accompany with a slice of toasted wholegrain bread ☑
- Chicken Noodle Soup (see recipe, p.211) served with 1 small wholegrain pitta bread, toasted
- Broccoli and Leek Soup (see recipe, p.210) served with a small granary roll ☑
- Chicken, Mushroom and Lemon Soup (see recipe, p.210) served with a small wholegrain roll (max. 150 kcal). Plus 1 pear or orange
- 1 pot Rosemary Conley Solo Slim Soup: choose from Tomato, Pea and Ham, Three Bean and Chorizo, Mushroom or Minestrone (order from www.rosemaryconley.com), plus 1 slice wholegrain bread and 1 piece fresh fruit

DINNERS

Chicken and turkey dinners

■ Chicken with Couscous: Season 1 × 120g skinless chicken breast with a little salt and plenty of freshly ground black pepper, then grill, steam or microwave. Serve with 1 blue Portion Pot® (50g uncooked weight) steamed couscous, plus unlimited salad or vegetables and 2 tsps Thai sweet chilli dipping sauce or mango chutney

■ 150g roast chicken breast (no skin) served with 100g dry-roast sweet potatoes plus 200g other vegetables of your choice (e.g. carrots, broccoli, cauliflower) and low-fat gravy

■ Quick and Easy Chicken Curry: Dry-fry 1 × 115g chopped chicken breast (no skin) in a preheated non-stick pan with ½ chopped onion and 1 crushed garlic clove. Sprinkle 1 tsp curry powder over and 'cook out' for 1 minute, then add 1 small chopped chilli, ½ chopped green pepper, 25g button mushrooms (optional) and 1 × 400g can chopped tomatoes, and simmer for 5 minutes to reduce. Serve with 1 blue Portion Pot® (55g uncooked weight) or 1 red Portion Pot® (144g cooked weight) basmati rice

■ Chicken in Mushroom Sauce: Dry-fry 100g chopped chicken breast (no skin) with ½ chopped onion and 6 button mushrooms. When the chicken is almost cooked, add 100g (⅓ can) Batchelors Low Fat Condensed Mushroom Soup, plus milk from allowance if needed to make a creamy sauce. Simmer until the chicken is completely cooked. Serve with 1 yellow Portion Pot® (100g) mashed sweet potato, plus other vegetables of your choice

■ Chinese Chicken Kebabs (see recipe, p.211) served with 1 blue Portion Pot® (55g uncooked weight) or 1 red Portion Pot® (144g cooked weight) basmati rice per person

■ Mixed Grill: 4 turkey rashers and 1 low-fat sausage, grilled, served with 1 dry-fried egg, 1 yellow Portion Pot® (115g) baked beans, unlimited grilled mushrooms plus 1 × 400g can tomatoes boiled well to reduce [P]

■ Barbecued Garlic Chicken (see recipe, p.212) served with 100g boiled new potatoes (with skins) plus salad or vegetables

■ Spicy Chicken Pasta: Dry-fry 110g chopped chicken breast (no skin) and ½ chopped onion in a non-stick wok and season with freshly ground black pepper. Add 1 crushed garlic clove, 1 sliced green pepper, 1 × 400g can chopped tomatoes, ½ small chopped chilli and a dash of Worcestershire sauce and allow to simmer for 5 minutes. Serve with 1 yellow Portion Pot® (45g uncooked weight) or 1 Portion Pot® (110g cooked weight) pasta shapes

■ Stir-Fry Chicken with Ginger: Chop 100g chicken breast (no skin) into bite-sized pieces and dry-fry in a non-stick pan with ½ crushed garlic clove. When the chicken has changed colour and is almost cooked through, add 1 chopped red or green pepper, 1 chopped celery stick, ½ chopped red onion, 25g mushrooms and 50g mangetout and dry-fry quickly but do not overcook. Just before serving add 1 tsp grated fresh ginger, soy sauce to taste and 1 tsp grated fresh coriander and heat through [P]

■ Southern Fried Turkey (see recipe, p.213) served hot with unlimited vegetables (excluding potatoes) or salad [P]

■ Chicken Shaslik (see recipe, p.212) served with 1 blue Portion Pot® (55g uncooked weight) or 1 red Portion Pot® (144g cooked weight) basmati rice per person

Beef dinners

■ 100g lean roast beef, thinly sliced, served with 100g dry-roasted potatoes and 200g other vegetables of your choice (excluding potatoes), plus low-fat gravy and 1 tsp horseradish sauce

■ Beef Kebabs: Cut 150g rump steak into bite-sized pieces and thread on to wooden skewers with 8 chestnut mushrooms, then baste with 50g tomato passata and 1 tsp balti curry paste. Cook the kebabs for 5–6 minutes in a health grill or 10 minutes under a conventional grill. Check the centre of meat is cooked and, when ready to serve, sprinkle with ½ tbsp chopped fresh coriander and serve with fresh green vegetables or salad [P]

■ Beef Fajitas: Dry-fry 120g sliced lean beef with ½ each sliced red and green pepper and ½ chopped red onion, then mix in 2 tsps fajita spice mix. Fill a low-fat tortilla wrap with the mixture and serve with 1 blue Portion Pot® (75g) tomato salsa and a large mixed salad tossed in oil-free dressing

- Steak in Mushroom Sauce: Dry-fry 2 thin beef steaks (250g total) quickly on both sides. Remove from the pan and keep warm. Add 100g chestnut mushrooms to the pan and cook for 1 minute before adding 1 tsp Knorr Touch of Taste beef stock and 75ml water. Bring the sauce to the boil and reduce by half. Remove from the heat and stir in ½ tbsp 3% fat yogurt. Transfer the steaks to a serving plate and top with the mushroom sauce. Serve with green vegetables or salad **P**
- 175g lean beef fillet or rump steak, grilled, served with a large salad plus 1 tbsp Hellmann's Extra Light Mayonnaise **P**
- Cheesy Cottage Pie (see recipe, p.214)
- Pasta Bolognese: Dry-fry 100g lean minced beef in a non-stick pan, seasoning well with black pepper. Drain off the fat, add ½ chopped onion, 1 crushed garlic clove and ½ chopped red pepper and dry-fry until soft. Stir in ¼ jar Dolmio Bolognese Original Light Pasta Sauce and 1 × 200g can chopped tomatoes and simmer for 10 minutes. Serve with 1 yellow Portion Pot® (45g uncooked weight) pasta shapes, boiled with a vegetable stock cube
- Baked Liver and Onions: Place 150g calves' liver in an ovenproof dish with 1 sliced onion. Cover with foil and cook in a moderate oven (180C, 350F, Gas Mark 4) for 15–20 minutes until lightly cooked. Make some low-fat gravy with gravy powder and add to the liver and onion. Serve with 1 yellow Portion Pot® (100g) mashed potato and other vegetables of your choice

Pork dinners

- 1 × 150g (raw weight) lean pork steak (all visible fat removed), grilled, served with 115g boiled new potatoes (with skins), 200g other vegetables of your choice, plus low-fat gravy and 1 tbsp apple sauce
- Spicy Pork Steak: Mix together 1 tsp ground cumin, 1 tsp ground ginger and 1 tsp smoked paprika on a plate, then press 300g lean pork steak into the spices and season with salt and pepper. Cook the steak in a health grill for 8–10 minutes or under a conventional grill for 8–10 minutes each side. Serve hot with a mixed salad or vegetables of your choice **P**
- Wine Braised Pork Slices (see recipe, p.215) served with 115g boiled new potatoes (with skins) and additional other vegetables of your choice

- Sweet and Sour Pork Chop: Grill 1 × 140g lean pork chop, all visible fat removed, and serve with 115g boiled new potatoes (with skins), 100g each carrots and broccoli, plus 1 yellow Portion Pot® (125ml) Uncle Ben's Sweet & Sour Light sauce
- 1 × 115g lean pork steak (all visible fat removed), grilled, served with 1 yellow Portion Pot® (100g) mashed sweet potato, plus unlimited other vegetables and low-fat gravy
- 3 low-fat pork sausages, grilled, served with 1 yellow Portion Pot® (100g) mashed, sweet potatoes plus unlimited vegetables and low-fat gravy
- Ham, Leek and Sweet Potato Pie (see recipe, p.216) served with unlimited vegetables (excluding potatoes) or salad
- Ham and Cheese Omelette: Beat 3 eggs with milk from allowance and cook in a non-stick pan. Add 25g grated Rosemary Conley low-fat Mature Cheese and 25g shredded ham. Serve with a large salad tossed in fat-free dressing **P**

Lamb dinners

- 1 × 150g lean lamb steak (raw weight), grilled, served with 115g boiled new potatoes (with skins), plus 200g other vegetables of your choice and a little low-fat gravy and mint sauce
- Lamb and Mushroom Goulash (see recipe, p.215) served with green vegetables
- Lamb Stir-Fry: Cut 150g lean lamb steak into strips and dry-fry with ½ chopped onion and ½ crushed garlic clove in a non-stick pan over a high heat for 1–2 minutes. Add 1 tsp mint sauce, 75g stir-fry vegetables and ½ tbsp soy sauce and toss well before cooking for 7–8 minutes. Serve on a bed of lightly cooked beansprouts **P**
- Lamb Medallions with Blackcurrant Sauce (see recipe, p.214) served with 100g boiled new potatoes (with skins) and unlimited vegetables

Fish and seafood dinners

- 150g cod fillet, microwaved or steamed, and 50g cooked prawns, served with ½ × 300g pack (150g) Schwartz for Fish low-fat Chunky Tomato, Olive and Rosemary Sauce, plus unlimited carrots and broccoli or courgettes and 1 yellow Portion Pot® (70g) peas **P**

■ 150g tuna steak, grilled, served with 1 blue Portion Pot® (50g uncooked weight) couscous (any flavour, e.g. see Ainsley Harriott range) plus 1 blue Portion Pot® (75g) tomato salsa and a large salad

■ Fish Pie: Place 50g each of fresh salmon, cod and shelled uncooked prawns in a small ovenproof dish and cover with ⅓ can Batchelors Low Fat Condensed Mushroom Soup, top with mashed potato (made by boiling 115g old potatoes then mashing with milk from allowance and seasoning well). Place in the oven and bake at 200C, 400F, Gas Mark 6 for 30 minutes or until the potato is browned on top. Serve with unlimited carrots and broccoli **P**

■ 1 × 115g (raw weight) salmon steak, steamed or microwaved, served with 80g boiled new potatoes (with skins), plus 1 yellow Portion Pot® (70g) frozen or canned peas, 100g steamed broccoli or asparagus and 1 tbsp Hellmann's Extra Light Mayonnaise

■ Oven-Baked Salmon: Place 1 × 110g salmon steak in an ovenproof dish, top with 1 tsp Thai sweet chilli dipping sauce and the juice of ½ lime. Bake in a preheated oven at 200C, 400F, Gas Mark 6 for 8–10 minutes, or until cooked. Serve with 100g boiled new potatoes (with skins) and unlimited green vegetables

■ Chilli Prawn Stir-Fry with Peppers and Mushrooms: Dry-fry 150g fresh prawns in a non-stick wok. When they have changed colour, add ½ each chopped red and green pepper, 5 button mushrooms, 1 chopped celery stick, ½ chopped red onion, 1 small courgette, chopped, and ½ pack of fresh (or 1 whole can) beansprouts. Do not overcook. Just before serving add 1 tbsp Thai sweet chilli dipping sauce and soy sauce to taste. Plus 1 low-fat yogurt or other low-fat dessert (max. 100 kcal and 5% fat) **P**

■ Prawn Saag (see recipe, p.217) served with 1 green Portion Pot® (170g) cooked egg noodles or 1 blue Portion Pot® (55g uncooked weight) or 1 red Portion Pot® (144g cooked weight) basmati rice per person. Plus 1 meringue nest topped with 1 tbsp 0% fat Greek yogurt and 2 sliced strawberries

■ Black Bean Prawns (see recipe, p.217) served with 1 blue Portion Pot® (55g uncooked weight) or 1 red Portion Pot® (144g cooked weight) basmati rice. Plus 1 Marks & Spencer meringue nest topped with 1 tsp 0% fat Greek yogurt and 1 tbsp raspberries

■ Chilli Prawn Stir-Fry with Asparagus: Dry-fry ½ chopped red onion and ½ crushed garlic clove in a non-stick pan until soft. Add 50g sliced asparagus and 100g uncooked, shelled prawns and continue cooking for 2–3 minutes. Pour in 1 × 75g pack chilli stir-fry sauce and stir well to coat the prawns and vegetables. Bring to the boil, then turn off the heat. Serve with salad and garnish with fresh chives **P**

Vegetarian dinners

■ Quorn Bolognese: Dry-fry 100g Quorn mince in a non-stick pan, seasoning well with black pepper. Add ½ chopped onion, 1 crushed garlic clove and ½ chopped red pepper and dry-fry until soft. Stir in ¼ jar Dolmio Bolognese Original Light Pasta Sauce and 1 × 200g can chopped tomatoes and simmer for 10 minutes. Serve with 1 yellow Portion Pot® (45g uncooked weight) pasta shapes, boiled with a vegetable stock cube **V**

■ Pasta Ratatouille: In a saucepan, mix together 1 small can of tomatoes, 2 tsps tomato purée, ½ chopped red onion, ½ chopped red or green pepper, ½ chopped aubergine and ½ sliced courgette. Sprinkle with 1 tsp oregano and some chopped fresh basil and simmer for 15–20 minutes, adding a little vegetable stock if required. When the vegetables are tender, mix in 1 red Portion Pot® (110g cooked weight) boiled pasta shapes and heat through **V**

■ Vegetable Chilli: Dry-fry 1 chopped onion in a preheated non-stick pan. Add 1 × 200g can mixed beans in chilli sauce and 1 × 200g can chopped tomatoes plus chopped vegetables (e.g. courgettes, mushrooms, carrots, peppers) and simmer for 15–20 minutes. Serve with 1 blue Portion Pot® (55g uncooked weight) or 1 red Portion Pot® (144g cooked weight) basmati rice **V**

■ 2 Quorn Lamb Style Grills, grilled, served with 115g boiled new potatoes (with skins), plus 200g other vegetables of your choice and a little low-fat gravy and mint sauce **V**

■ 1 × 200g oven-baked sweet potato topped with 200g baked beans and served with a side salad tossed in low-fat dressing of your choice **V**

■ 2 Quorn Peppered Steaks, grilled, served with a large salad plus 1 tbsp Hellmann's Extra Light Mayonnaise **V** **P**

■ Cheesy Quorn Bake: Dry-fry 1 finely chopped red onion and 1 crushed garlic clove in a non-stick pan until soft, then stir in 100g Quorn mince and cook for a further 2 minutes. Add 200g chopped tomatoes, 250g tomato passata, ½–1 tsp vegetable stock powder, ½ tbsp chives and reduce to a gentle simmer. While the Quorn mixture is simmering, heat a non-stick griddle pan and cook 150g chopped courgettes on both sides until lightly browned, seasoning with black pepper. Layer the courgettes and Quorn mixture in an ovenproof dish. Pour 150g 2% fat Greek yogurt over the top and add 25g grated Rosemary Conley low-fat Mature Cheese (or vegetarian alternative) and black pepper to taste. Bake in a preheated oven at 200C, 400F, Gas Mark 6 for 20 minutes until the cheese has melted and the dish is hot all the way through. Garnish with chopped chives ☑ P

■ Sweet and Sour Quorn: Dry-fry ½ × 350g pack Quorn Chicken Style Pieces (175g) with ½ chopped onion, ½ each chopped red and green pepper, 5 button mushrooms, halved, 1 chopped celery stick and 1 small chopped courgette. Add 1 yellow Portion Pot® (125ml) Uncle Ben's Sweet & Sour Light sauce and heat through before serving. Plus 1 low-fat yogurt or other dessert (max. 100 kcal and 5% fat) ☑ P

■ ½ pack any branded fresh filled pasta (max. 5% fat) served with ½ pot ready-made low-fat fresh tomato-based sauce (max. 400 kcal total for whole meal) ☑

■ Chilli Quorn Stir-Fry with Asparagus: Dry-fry ½ chopped red onion and ½ crushed garlic clove in a non-stick pan until soft. Add 50g sliced asparagus and 100g Quorn pieces and continue cooking for 2–3 minutes. Pour in 1 × 75g pack chilli stir-fry sauce and stir well to coat the Quorn pieces and the vegetables. Bring to the boil, then turn off the heat. Serve with salad and garnish with fresh chives ☑ P

■ Quorn and Rice Bake (see recipe, p.220) served with unlimited vegetables (excluding potatoes) ☑

■ 1 low-fat veggie burger (max. 180 kcal and 5% fat, e.g. Grassington's Vegetable Quarter Pounder or Quorn Quarter Pounder) cooked as per instructions. Serve with 115g boiled new potatoes (with skins) and a large salad tossed in low-fat dressing ☑

■ 2 Quorn sausages, grilled, served with ½ pack readymade cauliflower cheese (max. 200 kcal and 5% fat) and green vegetables of your choice ☑

■ 3 Quorn sausages, grilled, served with 1 yellow Portion Pot® (100g) mashed sweet potatoes, plus unlimited other vegetables and a little low-fat gravy ☑

■ Pasta with Tomato and Basil Sauce: Mix 1 red Portion Pot® (80g uncooked weight) or 1 green Portion Pot® (176g cooked weight) boiled pasta shapes with ½ jar (approx. 200g) ready-made tomato and basil pasta sauce and heat through. Serve with chopped fresh basil leaves and a sprinkling of Parmesan shavings, plus a large green salad tossed in fat-free dressing ☑

■ Roasted Pepper Pasta (see recipe, p.219) served with a large salad tossed in fat-free dressing ☑

■ Leek and Sage Meatballs with Pasta (see recipe, p.218) ☑

■ Cauliflower Bhaji (see recipe, p.221) served with 1 blue Portion Pot® (55g uncooked weight) or 1 red Portion Pot® (144g cooked weight) basmati rice per person ☑

■ Any low-fat vegetarian ready meal (max. 400 kcal and 5% fat, including any accompaniments) ☑

Ready meals

■ 1 × 400g pack Asda Good For You Chilli Beef & Mushrooms. Serve with green salad tossed in fat-free dressing

■ 1 × 400g pack Asda Good For You Spicy Tomato Chicken. Plus 1 low-fat yogurt (max. 120 kcal and 5% fat)

■ 1 × 400g pack Asda Good For You Chicken Chasseur. Serve with unlimited vegetables (excluding potatoes)

■ 1 × 450g pack Asda Good For You Chicken Tikka Masala & Pilau Rice

■ 1 × 400g pack Sainsbury's Be Good To Yourself Chicken Tikka Masala with Pilau Rice

■ 1 × 400g pack Sainsbury's Be Good To Yourself Lasagne. Serve with green salad tossed in fat-free dressing

■ 1 × 400g pack Sainsbury's Be Good To Yourself Chicken and Pasta Bake. Serve with green salad tossed in fat-free dressing

- 1 × 400g pack Asda Good For You Chicken & Broccoli. Serve with unlimited green vegetables
- 1 × 375g pack Morrisons Eat Smart Diet Chicken in Peppercorn Sauce with Sliced Roast Potatoes. Serve with unlimited green vegetables
- 1 × 375g pack Morrisons Chicken in Tomato and Basil Sauce. Serve with unlimited vegetables (excluding potatoes)
- 1 × 400g pack Morrisons Eat Smart Chicken Korma with Pilau Rice
- Marks & Spencer Count On Us Steak Yorkshires (1 pudding per person). Serve with 100g lean roast beef and unlimited green vegetables and low-fat gravy
- 1 × 400g pack Marks & Spencer Count On Us Cajun Chicken Fettucine. Serve with green salad tossed in fat-free dressing
- 1 × 400g pack Marks & Spencer Count On Us Braised Beef in Ale. Serve with green vegetables.
- 1 × 400g pack Marks & Spencer Count on Us King Prawn Masala. Serve with green salad tossed in fat-free dressing
- 1 × 400g pack Waitrose Low Saturated Fat Chicken & Asparagus with Roast Potatoes
- 1 × 395g pack Waitrose Low Saturated Fat Chicken Korma with Pilau Rice
- Any meal from Rosemary Conley's Solo Slim range (order from www.rosemaryconley.com):
  - 1 × 300g pack Rosemary Conley Solo Slim Beef Meatballs and Potato. Serve with unlimited vegetables (excluding potatoes)
  - 1 × 300g pack Rosemary Conley Solo Slim Lamb Hotpot. Plus 1 low-fat yogurt (max. 150 kcal and 5% fat)
  - 1 × 300g pack Rosemary Conley Solo Slim Chilli and Rice. Serve with 1 × 50g crusty wholegrain roll or small wholemeal pitta bread
  - 1 × 300g pack Rosemary Conley Solo Slim Spicy Vegetable and Lentil Dahl. Plus 1 low-fat yogurt (max. 150 kcal and 5% fat) ☑

POWER SNACKS

Fruit
- 1 whole papaya, peeled and deseeded ☑
- 100g cherries ☑
- 75g fresh mango ☑
- 12 seedless grapes ☑
- 1 medium pear ☑
- 100g fresh pineapple ☑
- 1 × 200g slice melon (weighed without skin) ☑
- 150g strawberries ☑
- 1 small apple ☑
- 2 kiwi fruit ☑
- 2 dried apricots ☑
- 20g sultanas ☑
- 1 kid's fun-size mini banana ☑
- 1 kiwi fruit plus 5 seedless grapes ☑
- 2 satsumas ☑
- 2 plums ☑
- ½ grapefruit sprinkled with 1 tsp sugar ☑
- 150g fresh fruit salad ☑
- 1 red Portion Pot® (115g) raspberries plus 50g strawberries ☑
- 1 yellow Portion Pot® (70g) blueberries plus 1 tsp low-fat natural yogurt ☑
- 1 yellow Portion Pot® (125ml) fresh orange or apple juice ☑
- 1 red Portion Pot® (115g) raspberries topped with 2 tsps low-fat yogurt (max. 5% fat) ☑
- 1 × 90g pack Tesco Fresh Apple and Grape Snack Pack ☑
- 100g any stewed fruit sweetened with low-cal sweetener ☑

Sweet
- 1 fat-free yogurt, any flavour (max. 50 kcal) ☑
- 1 Hartley's Low Calorie Jelly topped with 1 tbsp Total 2% Greek Yoghurt and 3 berries of your choice
- 1 blue Portion Pot® (14g) Special K (eat dry or with milk from allowance) ☑
- 1 Caxton Pink 'n' Whites wafer ☑

Savoury
- 1 rice cake spread with 20g Philadelphia Extra Light soft cheese and sliced cucumber ☑

- 5 mini low-fat bread sticks plus 1 tsp (25g) Total 0 % fat Greek Yoghurt mixed with chopped chives ☑
- 1 Asda Good For You Chicken Noodle Cup Soup
- 10 sweet silverskin pickled onions plus 10 cherry tomatoes ☑
- 20g low-fat cheese (max. 5 % fat) plus 5 cherry tomatoes ☑
- 1 Rakusen's cracker topped with 1 × 20g triangle Laughing Cow Extra Light soft cheese, plus 5 cherry tomatoes
- 1 Ryvita spread thinly with Philadelphia Extra Light soft cheese ☑
- 1 Ryvita, spread with Marmite and topped with 2 tsps low-fat cottage cheese ☑
- 1 blue Portion Pot® (75g) tomato salsa plus 1 carrot, 1 celery stick and 1 × 5cm piece cucumber sliced into crudités ☑
- 2 carrots, cut into sticks, served with 1 tbsp low-fat yogurt mixed with fresh chopped chives and finely chopped red onion ☑
- 10 cherry tomatoes, plus chunks of carrots, cucumber and green or red pepper ☑
- 1 small bowl of mixed salad tossed in fat-free dressing ☑

DESSERTS

All the following desserts are less than 5 % fat.

Ice cream and iced desserts
- Strawberry and Rhubarb Mousse (see recipe, p.223) **125 kcal**
- 1 × 100ml serving Asda Triple Chocolate Dairy Ice Cream **101 kcal**
- 1 × 60g serving Tesco Healthy Living Banoffee Frozen Dessert **92 kcal**
- 1 × 100ml serving Wall's Soft Scoop Raspberry Ripple flavour ice cream **82 kcal** ☑
- 1 × 70g pot Marks & Spencer Count On Us Raspberry Mousse **80 kcal**
- 1 × 70g pot Marks & Spencer Count On Us Chocolate Mousse **80 kcal**
- 1 The Skinny Cow Triple Chocolate Stick **78 kcal** ☑
- 1 × 100ml serving Carte D'Or Lemon Sorbet **78 kcal**
- Tropical Sorbet (see recipe, p.222) **74 kcal** ☑
- 1 × 100ml serving Carte D'Or Light Vanilla ice cream **70 kcal**
- 1 × 100ml serving Wall's Soft Scoop Light Vanilla flavour ice cream **62 kcal**

Fruit, meringues and jelly
- Coffee and Apricot Roulade (see recipe, p.223) **108 kcal**
- 150g fresh fruit salad plus 1 tsp low-fat yogurt **100 kcal**
- Eton Mess: Break up 1 Marks & Spencer meringue basket and mix with 1 tbsp 0 % fat Greek yogurt and 1 large chopped strawberry **99 kcal** ☑
- 1 Marks & Spencer meringue nest filled with 1 tbsp 0 % fat Greek yogurt and topped with 1 tbsp fresh raspberries or blueberries **90 kcal** ☑
- 1 Marks & Spencer meringue basket filled with 1 tsp 0 % fat Greek yogurt and topped with 1 slice pineapple, chopped **85 kcal** ☑
- 1 × 120g pot Del Monte Fruitini Fruit Pieces in juice **71 kcal** ☑
- 1 Hartley's Low Sugar Jelly plus 1 piece any fresh fruit **60 kcal**

Yogurts and fromage frais
- 1 × 200g pot Müllerlight Apricot fat free yogurt **98 kcal**
- 1 × 200g pot Müllerlight Wild Blueberry fat free yogurt **94 kcal**
- 1 × 55g pot Asda Great Fruity Stuff fromage frais, any flavour **94 kcal** ☑
- 1 × 125g pot Yeo Valley Organic Low Fat Raspberry Yogurt **94 kcal** ☑
- 1 × 150g Asda Good For You Rhubarb Yogurt **91 kcal** ☑
- 1 pot Tesco Healthy Living Lemon Cheesecake yogurt **90 kcal** ☑
- 1 × 165g pot Müllerlight Vanilla Yogurt sprinkled with Dark Chocolate **86 kcal**
- 1 × 125g pot Sainsbury's Be Good To Yourself Blueberry & Cranberry Fruit Yogurt **86 kcal**
- 1 × 120g pot Danone Shape Fat Free Feel Fuller For Longer yogurt, any flavour **75 kcal** ☑

Puddings and cakes
- Crunchy Apple and Blackberry Pie (see recipe, p.225) **139 kcal** ☑
- Plum Tatin (see recipe, p.224) **107 kcal**
- 1 × 100ml serving Morrisons Absolutely Gorgeous Toffee Pecan Temptation **102 kcal**
- Banana Muffins (see recipe, p.224) **99 kcal**
- 1 Sainsbury's Lemon Cake Slice **97 kcal** ☑
- 1 Asda Good For You Lemon Slice **97 kcal** ☑
- 1 Asda Good for You Cherry Bakewell Slice **96 kcal**
- 1 Asda Good For You Chocolate Slice **95 kcal** ☑
- 1 Mr Kipling Delightful Apple Slice **91 kcal** ☑
- 1 Asda Good for You Carrot and Orange Cake Slice **77 kcal**
- 1 × 100g serving Tesco Healthy Eating Summer Fruits Pudding **72 kcal**
- 1 × ⅛ slice Soreen Lincolnshire Plum Fruit Loaf **65 kcal** ☑

TREATS

If you wish, you can combine one or more lower calorie treats. You can also save up your treats over seven days for a bigger treat or a special occasion.

HIGH-FAT TREATS FOR 100 KCAL OR LESS
All the following treats are more than 5% fat.

Crisps
- 10 Pringles Lights Sour Cream & Onion flavour **99 kcal** ☑
- 1 × 21g bag Boots Shapers Salt & Vinegar Chipsticks **99 kcal** ☑
- 1 × 25g bag Walkers Baked Salt & Vinegar crisps **98 kcal** ☑
- 1 × 25g bag Jacob's Original Twiglets **96 kcal** ☑
- 1 × 18g bag Walkers Baked Wotsits Really Cheesy **95 kcal** ☑
- 1 × 19g bag Cheese & Onion Flavour Pom-Bear Teddy-shaped Potato Snacks **95 kcal** ☑
- 1 × 25g bag Walkers Squares Cheese & Onion Flavour Potato Snack **95 kcal** ☑
- 1 × 21g bag Golden Wonder Golden Lights Sour Cream & Onion crisps **94 kcal** ☑
- 1 × 21g bag Sainsbury's Be Good To Yourself 35% Less Fat Salt & Black Pepper Light & Crunchy Snacks **94 kcal** ☑
- 1 × 23g bag Walkers French Fries Ready Salted **94 kcal** ☑
- 1 × 25g bag Walkers Squares Ready Salted **94 kcal** ☑
- 1 × 24g bag Kettle Crispy Bakes Mild Cheese with Sweet Onion **91 kcal** ☑
- 1 × 18g bag Skips Prawn Cocktail snacks **89 kcal**
- 1 × 18g bag Walkers Quavers Cheese Flavour **87 kcal** ☑

Cereal bars and cakes
- 1 Cadbury Highlights Toffee Flavour Cake Bar **95 kcal** ☑
- 1 Mr Kipling Delightful Chocolate Cake Slice **95 kcal** ☑
- 1 Harvest Chewee White Choc Chip Cereal Bar **94 kcal** ☑

- 1 Kellogg's Special K Bar **90 kcal** ☑
- 1 Kellogg's Coco Pops Cereal & Milk Bar **85 kcal** ☑

Biscuits
- 2 Weight Watchers Raspberry & White Chocolate Cookies **98 kcal** ☑
- 2 Weight Watchers Double Choc Chip Cookies **98 kcal** ☑
- 3 Bahlsen Deloba biscuits **98 kcal** ☑
- 2 Sainsbury's Taste The Difference Belgian Chocolate Biscuit Thins **96 kcal**
- 1 Marks & Spencer All Butter Fruity Flapjack Cookie **95 kcal** ☑
- 3 Fox's Party Rings **93 kcal** ☑
- 2 McVitie's Jaffa Cakes **92 kcal** ☑
- 1 McVitie's Dark Chocolate HobNob **92 kcal** ☑
- 3 Rombouts Café Biscuits **92 kcal**
- 3 Cadbury Milk Chocolate Fingers **90 kcal** ☑
- 3 Lotus Original Caramelised Biscuits **90 kcal** ☑
- 1 Marks & Spencer Dutch Shortcake **90 kcal**
- 1 McVitie's Moments Chocolate Viennese Melt **90 kcal**
- 1 Tesco All Butter Traditional Scottish Shortbread Finger **90 kcal** ☑
- 4 Asda Rich Tea Fingers **88 kcal** ☑
- 1 Tesco Free From Golden Crunch biscuit **85 kcal** ☑
- 1 McVitie's Belgian Chocolate Chunk Boaster **86 kcal** ☑
- 1 Jammie Dodgers Original **83 kcal** ☑
- 1 McVitie's Milk Chocolate Mint Digestives **81 kcal**
- 1 Green & Black's Organic Chocolate Flapjack biscuit **80 kcal** ☑
- 4 Cadbury Snaps (any flavour) **80 kcal** ☑
- 1 McVitie's Light Milk Chocolate Digestive **78 kcal** ☑
- 1 Fox's Golden Crunch Creams **75 kcal** ☑

Sweets and chocolate
- 4 Bassetts Murray Mints **100 kcal** ☑
- 1 Boots Shapers Crispy Caramel Bar **99 kcal**
- 1 × 20g fun size bag M & Ms **98 kcal**
- 1 fun-size Twix **98 kcal**
- 1 Tesco Value Choc Ice **95 kcal**
- 2 segments Terry's Chocolate Orange **90 kcal** ☑
- 6 Cadbury Mini Eggs **90 kcal** ☑
- 1 fun-size Mars Bar **88 kcal**

- 1 mini bag Nestlé Milkybar Buttons **87 kcal**
- 1 Thorntons Mini Caramel Shortcake **86 kcal** ☑
- 4 Werther's Original **84 kcal** ☑
- 2 Galaxy Mini Eggs **80 kcal** ☑
- 1 Ferrero Rocher **75 kcal** ☑
- 1 Thorntons Continental Chocolate **70 kcal** ☑

LOW-FAT TREATS FOR 100 KCAL OR LESS
All the following treats are less than 5 % fat.

Sweet treats
- 2 Caxton Pink 'n' Whites **100 kcal** ☑
- 5 Bassetts Jelly Babies **100 kcal**
- 25 Jelly Belly Jelly Beans **100 kcal**
- 10 Maynards Wine Gums Light **100 kcal**
- 24 Skittles **97 kcal** ☑
- 1 × 28g treat bag Rowntree's Jelly Tots **96 kcal** ☑
- 4 Bassetts Liquorice Allsorts **91 kcal**
- 5 Starburst Twisted Chews **90 kcal** ☑
- 5 Haribo Tangfastics **85 kcal**

Savoury treats
- 1 × 25g bag Sainsbury's Be Good To Yourself Sea Salt & Cracked Black Pepper Pretzel Sticks **95 kcal**
- 1 × 25g pack Marks & Spencer Mini Salted Pretzels **94 kcal**
- 1 × 30g bag Ryvita Minis Salt & Vinegar **93 kcal**
- 1 × 25g bag Morrisons Eat Smart Sea Salt Pretzels **87 kcal**
- 1 × 25g bag Marks & Spencer Count On Us Sour Cream & Chive Baked Potato Crisps **85 kcal**
- 1 × 25g bag Marks & Spencer Count On Us Lightly Salted Baked Potato Crisps **85 kcal**
- 1 × 20g pack Asda Good For You Crispy Cracker Selection Hickory Smoked Barbecue Flavour **76 kcal**
- 1 × 20g pack Asda Good For You Crispy Cracker Selection Sun-Dried Tomato and Herb Flavour **76 kcal**
- 1 × 20g pack Asda Good For You Crispy Cracker Selection Thai Style Sweet Chilli Flavour **76 kcal**
- 1 × 25g bag Marks & Spencer Count On Us Smokey Bacon Potato Hoops **60 kcal**
- 1 × 18g pack Ryvita Limbos Cheese & Onion **63 kcal** ☑
- 1 × 18g pack Ryvita Limbos Smokey Bacon **63 kcal** ☑
- 1 × 18g pack Ryvita Limbos Salt & Vinegar **62 kcal** ☑

ALCOHOLIC DRINKS

In Phases 2 and 3 you are allowed an alcoholic drink each day up to 100 calories. Use Slimline and low-calorie mixers with spirits to keep the calories down. Here is a quick guide to calories.

Beer and cider (per 300ml/½ pint)
Bitter 91 kcal
Cider (dry) 100 kcal
Guinness 90 kcal
Lager 82 kcal

Brandy and liqueurs (per 25ml measure)
Brandy 50 kcal
Cointreau 78 kcal
Grand Marnier 78 kcal
Southern Comfort 81 kcal
Tia Maria 75 kcal

Sprits (per 25ml measure)
Bacardi 56 kcal
Gin 50 kcal
Rum 50 kcal
Vodka 50 kcal
Whisky 50 kcal

Vermouth (per 50ml measure)
Martini Extra Dry 48 kcal
Martini Rosso 70 kcal

Wine and fortified wine (per yellow Portion Pot®/125ml)
Champagne 95 kcal
Red wine 85 kcal
Rosé wine (medium) 89 kcal
White wine (dry) 83 kcal
White wine (medium) 93 kcal

Fortified wine (per 50ml measure)
Dry sherry 58 kcal
Sweet sherry 68 kcal
Port 79 kcal

Recipes

SOUPS

Broccoli and Leek Soup ✓❄

SERVES 4
Per serving
68 calories 1.9g fat
Preparation 10 minutes
Cooking time 20 minutes

4 leeks, sliced
2 garlic cloves, crushed
1 tsp chopped fresh thyme
1 litre vegetable stock
200g broccoli florets
2 tbsps chopped fresh parsley
200ml semi-skimmed milk
2 tbsps virtually fat free fromage frais
salt and freshly ground black pepper

1   Place the leeks, garlic and thyme in a large saucepan. Add the stock and bring to the boil. Simmer gently for 15 minutes.
2   Stir in the broccoli and parsley and continue cooking until the broccoli is tender.
3   Allow to cool a little, then pour into a liquidiser, add the milk and blend until smooth. Return to the saucepan to reheat, adding more seasoning if required.
4   Just before serving, remove from the heat and stir in the fromage frais.

☑ means suitable for vegetarians
❄ means suitable for freezing

Chicken, Mushroom and Lemon Soup

SERVES 4
Per serving
141 calories 2.7g fat
Preparation 10 minutes
Cooking 20 minutes

1 × 150g skinless chicken breast, cut into small pieces
2 celery sticks, finely chopped
2 leeks, finely chopped
2 garlic cloves, crushed
300ml vegetable stock
10g dried mushrooms
300ml semi-skimmed milk
1 tbsp cornflour
1 tsp fine lemon zest
1 tbsp chopped fresh parsley
2 tbsps low-fat yogurt
fresh chives to serve

1   Preheat a large non-stick pan, then dry-fry the chicken, celery, leeks and garlic for 2–3 minutes. Stir in the stock and mushrooms and boil until the mushrooms are soft.
2   Pour the milk into the soup and simmer gently for 10–15 minutes.
3   Mix the cornflour with a little cold water and stir into the soup, along with the lemon zest, to allow the soup to thicken.
4   Once the soup has thickened, stir in the parsley. Just before serving, remove from the heat and stir in the yogurt. Garnish with a few chives.

TIP Dried mushrooms add a strong flavour to this creamy soup

Chicken Noodle Soup ❄

SERVES 4
Per serving
170 calories 1.4g fat
Preparation 25 minutes
Cooking 30 minutes

200g lean chicken breast (no skin), cut into strips
3 baby leeks, finely chopped
1 garlic clove, crushed
2 tsps ground coriander
½ tsp ground turmeric
1 small fresh green chilli, chopped
seeds from 4 crushed cardamom pods
600ml vegetable stock
100g fine rice noodles
2 tbsps chopped fresh basil
50g shredded fresh watercress
freshly ground black pepper

1   Preheat a non-stick wok or frying pan, then dry-fry the chicken until lightly browned on all sides and season with black pepper. Place to one side.
2   Place the leeks, garlic, spices, vegetable stock and rice noodles in a large saucepan and bring to a gentle simmer.
3   When the noodles are cooked, add the chicken to the pan and stir in the basil and watercress. Serve straight away.

TIP Using rice noodles makes this a gluten-free dish

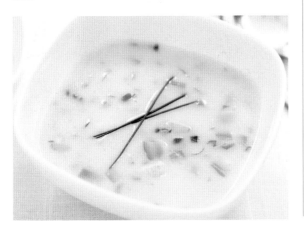

CHICKEN AND TURKEY

Chinese Chicken Kebabs

SERVES 2
Per serving
204 calories 1.6g fat
Preparation 10 minutes
Marinating 1 hour
Cooking 20 minutes

2 medium-sized skinless chicken breasts
1 red pepper, diced
1 small can water chestnuts
1 tbsp dark brown sugar
1 tbsp cider vinegar
1 tsp finely chopped fresh ginger
1 tbsp tomato purée
salt and freshly ground black pepper
chopped spring onions to serve

1   Cut the chicken into chunks. Thread the chicken, red pepper and water chestnuts on to 4 wooden or metal skewers and place on a baking tray. Season with salt and black pepper.
2   Mix together the remaining ingredients, then drizzle over the kebabs. Leave the kebabs for at least an hour to allow them to absorb the marinade.
3   Cook the kebabs in a health grill for 10 minutes or under a preheated hot grill for 8–10 minutes each side.
4   Transfer to serving plates and garnish with spring onion.

TIP Marinate the kebabs overnight for maximum flavour

◀ *Chicken Mushroom and Lemon Soup*

Barbecued Garlic Chicken

SERVES 4
Per serving
155 calories 1.4g fat
Preparation 10 minutes
Marinating 1 hour
Cooking 30 minutes

4 skinless chicken breasts (400g total)
salt and freshly ground black pepper

for the marinade
2 tbsps sweet chilli sauce
2 tbsps runny honey
1 tbsp Worcestershire sauce
2 garlic cloves, peeled and chopped
1 red onion, finely chopped
pinch of fennel seeds

1 Combine the marinade ingredients in a mixing
   bowl.
2 Season the chicken breasts with salt and black
   pepper and place in the bottom of an ovenproof
   dish. Spoon the marinade over the chicken and
   leave to marinate for at least 1 hour.
3 Cook under a preheated grill or on a preheated
   barbecue for 25–30 minutes until cooked through
   to the centre.
5 Serve straight away with a selection of fresh
   vegetables or salads.

*TIP For maximum flavour, leave the chicken to
marinate overnight in the refrigerator*

Chicken Shaslik

SERVES 4
Per serving
170 calories 2.4g fat
Preparation 15 minutes
Cooking 30 minutes

4 skinless chicken breasts (400g total)
1 red pepper, cut into chunks
1 green pepper, cut into chunks
1 red onion, cut into chunks
2 garlic cloves, crushed
1 × 2cm piece fresh ginger, peeled and chopped
1 tsp ground turmeric
2 tsps ground coriander
2 tsps tandoori powder
1 × 400g can chopped tomatoes
1–2 tsps vegetable stock powder
salt and freshly ground black pepper

1 Preheat a non-stick wok.
2 Chop the chicken breasts into chunks.
3 Dry-fry the peppers and onion in the wok for 2–3
   minutes. Add the chicken, garlic and ginger and
   cook until the chicken is sealed. Stir in the spices
   and cook for a further minute. Finally, add the
   tomatoes and stock powder, then reduce the heat
   and simmer gently for 10 minutes before serving.
4 For a dinner option, serve with1 blue Portion Pot®
   (55g uncooked weight) or 1 red Portion Pot®
   (144g cooked weight) basmati rice per person.

*TIP Mix together some chopped fresh
coriander and a little low-fat yogurt to make a
simple sauce to serve alongside this dish*

Southern Fried Turkey

SERVES 2
Per serving
354 calories 6.2 g fat
Preparation 10 minutes
Cooking 30 minutes

4 thin turkey escalopes (320g total)
1 egg, beaten

for the coating
4 tbsps granary breadcrumbs
1 garlic clove, crushed
1 tsp paprika
1 tsp jerk seasoning
1 tbsp chopped fresh chives
salt and freshly ground black pepper

1 Preheat the oven to 200C, 400F, Gas Mark 6.
2 Mix together the breadcrumbs, garlic and
   seasonings and transfer to a non-stick baking tray.
   Place in the oven for 10 minutes until the
   breadcrumbs are lightly toasted.
3 Dip the turkey escalopes in the beaten egg and
   then the breadcrumbs and place on a non-stick
   baking tray. Bake in the oven for 25–30 minutes
   until cooked through.
4 Serve with fresh vegetables or salad.

Turkey and Mango Samosas

SERVES 4
Per serving
227 calories 6.1g fat
Preparation 20 minutes
Cooking 15–20 minutes

2 baby leeks, finely chopped
1 garlic clove, crushed
200g turkey mince
1–2 tsps vegetable stock powder
1 tbsp chopped fresh mint
1 tbsp mango chutney
4 sheets filo pastry
olive oil spray
salt and freshly ground black pepper

1 Preheat the oven to 200C, 400F, Gas Mark 6.
2 Preheat a non-stick frying pan, then dry-fry the
   leeks and garlic for 2–3 minutes until soft. Add the
   turkey and continue cooking for 5 minutes. Stir in
   the stock powder, mint and chutney and mix well.
   Remove from the heat and allow to cool.
3 Place the filo sheets on a chopping board. Cut each
   sheet into 3 lengthways, then lightly spray with oil
   spray. Place a dessertspoon of turkey mixture at
   each end of the strips, fold the pastry over
   diagonally to enclose the meat in a triangle, then
   transfer to a baking tray and spray again with oil.
4 Bake in the oven for 15–20 minutes until golden
   brown. Serve with fresh vegetables or salad.

*TIP These tasty pastry triangles also make
ideal party food*

BEEF, LAMB AND PORK

Lamb Medallions with Blackcurrant Sauce

SERVES 4
Per serving
200 calories 10.8g fat
Preparation 10 minutes
Marinating 30 minutes
Cooking 15 minutes

8 lamb medallions, all visible fat removed
1 tbsp blackcurrant jelly
2 garlic cloves, crushed
150ml vegetable stock
1 tbsp chopped fresh mint
salt and freshly ground black pepper

1 Place the lamb in a shallow dish and season with salt and pepper.
2 In a small saucepan heat together the blackcurrant jelly, garlic and vegetable stock for 2 minutes until the garlic is soft. Allow to cool, then stir in the mint.
3 Drizzle the sauce over the lamb and leave to marinate for 30 minutes.
4 Preheat the grill to high. Place the lamb on a baking tray and cook under the hot grill for 4–5 minutes each side, turning regularly. Serve hot.
5 For a dinner option, serve with 100g boiled new potatoes (with skins) and unlimited vegetables per person.

TIP Lamb medallions are the leanest cut of lamb available and they can be cooked and eaten pink

Cheesy Cottage Pie ❄

SERVES 4
Per serving
409 calories 16.3g fat
Preparation 10 minutes
Cooking 40 minutes

300g celeriac, peeled and chopped
300g sweet potato, peeled and chopped
500g lean beef mince
1 red onion, finely chopped
2 garlic cloves, crushed
2 tsps vegetable stock powder
3 carrots (300g total), peeled and diced
1 tbsp chopped fresh herbs
1 tbsp gravy granules
2 tbsps skimmed milk
50g Rosemary Conley low-fat Mature Cheese, grated
salt and freshly ground black pepper

1 Preheat the oven to 200C, 400F, Gas Mark 6. Preheat a non-stick pan.
2 Boil the celeriac and potatoes together in a saucepan of water until soft.
3 Meanwhile, dry-fry the mince in the non-stick pan until lightly browned. Tip the mince into a sieve to drain off the fat, then return it to the pan, add the onion, garlic and stock powder and cook for 3–4 minutes.
4 Add the carrots and herbs to the pan, then pour in 300ml water and bring to a gentle simmer. Add the gravy granules and continue to simmer for 20 minutes to allow the sauce to thicken. Check the seasoning, then transfer to an ovenproof dish.
5 Drain the celeriac and potatoes and mash well, adding the skimmed milk and seasoning with salt and black pepper. Spread the potato mixture over the meat and vegetables and smooth over the top, using a fork. Finally sprinkle the cheese on top.
6 Bake in the top of the oven for 20 minutes until golden brown.

TIP Using half sweet potatoes and mashed celeriac lowers the Gi rating of this dish

Lamb and Mushroom Goulash ❄

SERVES 4
Per serving
332 calories 10.6g fat
Preparation 10 minutes
Cooking 70 minutes

2 red onions, diced
2 garlic cloves, crushed
450g lean diced lamb
1 tbsp flour
2 tsps paprika
1.2 litres meat stock
10g dried wild mushrooms
2 tbsps tomato purée
450g small new potatoes
2 celery sticks, chopped
200g button mushrooms
1 tbsp mixed herbs (e.g. parsley, thyme, chives)
salt and freshly ground black pepper

1 Preheat a non-stick pan, then dry-fry the onions and garlic until the onion starts to brown.
2 Add the lamb to the pan, season with salt and black pepper and cook until sealed. Sprinkle the flour and paprika over and cook out for 1 minute, then gradually stir in the meat stock.
3 Add the remaining ingredients, then cover and simmer gently for 1 hour until the meat is tender. Serve with green vegetables.

TIP Choose lean diced lamb and remove all visible traces of fat before cooking

Wine Braised Pork Slices ❄

SERVES 4
Per serving
191 calories 4.5g fat
Preparation 10 minutes
Cooking 25 minutes

1 red onion, diced
2 garlic cloves, crushed
4 lean pork slices (400g total), all visible fat removed
100g chestnut mushrooms, sliced
2 tsps ground coriander
75ml red wine
1–2 tsps vegetable stock powder
2 × 400g cans chopped tomatoes
salt and freshly ground black pepper
fresh parsley to garnish

1 Preheat a non-stick pan, then dry-fry the onion and garlic until the onion is lightly browned.
2 Add the pork slices to the pan and cook until sealed, seasoning with salt and black pepper. Stir in the mushrooms and coriander and cook, mixing well, before adding the vegetable stock powder and tomatoes. Cover and simmer for 20 minutes until the sauce has reduced.
3 Transfer to serving plates and garnish with fresh parsley.
4 For a dinner option, serve with 115g boiled new potatoes (with skins) per person and additional other vegetables of your choice.

Wine Braised Pork Slices ▶

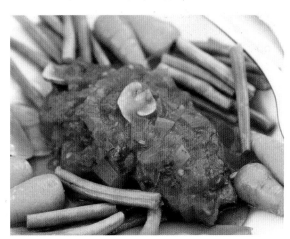

Ham, Leek and Sweet Potato Pie ❄

SERVES 4
Per serving
303 calories 3.5g fat
Preparation 10 minutes
Cooking 20 minutes

900g sweet potatoes, peeled
2 leeks, washed and sliced
100g thin ham, chopped
2–3 tbsps semi-skimmed milk
100g low-fat mature cheese
pinch of nutmeg
4 medium-sized tomatoes
salt and freshly ground black pepper

1 Preheat the oven to 200C, 400F, Gas Mark 6.
2 Boil the potatoes in a large pan of salted water until soft. Drain the potatoes, then mash them, adding the leeks, ham and milk.
3 Using a wooden spoon, fold in half the cheese along with the nutmeg and season to taste with salt and black pepper, then pile the potato mixture into an ovenproof dish.
4 Slice the tomatoes and arrange on top of the potatoes. Sprinkle with the remaining cheese and bake in the oven for 20 minutes or until golden brown.
5 Serve with fresh vegetables (excluding potatoes) or salad.

TIP If you slice the leeks very fine, they will not need pre-cooking before adding to the potatoes

Brunch Pitta

MAKES 2
Per pitta
291 calories 6.1g fat
Preparation 5 minutes
Cooking 10 minutes

2 pitta breads (max. 200 calories each)
4 rashers lean back bacon
2 tomatoes, sliced in half
2 large mushrooms (50g total), sliced
1 tbsp tomato ketchup
freshly ground black pepper

1 Preheat a health grill or conventional grill to high.
2 Cook the bacon, tomatoes and mushrooms in the health grill for 4–5 minutes or place in a grill tray or on a baking tray and cook under the conventional grill for 4–5 minutes each side, turning regularly. Remove and keep warm.
3 Warm the pittas in the health grill or under the conventional grill for 1 minute until puffed up, then split them in half and spread the insides with the ketchup. Divide the bacon, tomatoes and mushrooms between the 2 pitta breads, then cut each pitta bread in half and serve.

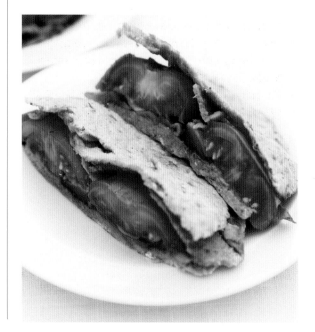

FISH AND SEAFOOD

Black Bean Prawns

SERVES 4
Per serving
135 calories 1.7g fat
Preparation 10 minutes
Cooking 10 minutes

2 red onions, finely sliced
2 garlic cloves, crushed
1 green and 1 red pepper, deseeded and sliced
110g chestnut mushrooms, sliced
200g fresh peeled prawns
100g Chinese cabbage, shredded
150ml black bean sauce
2 tbsps low-salt soy sauce
1 tbsp maple syrup
zest and juice of 1 lemon
freshly ground black pepper

1 Preheat a non-stick wok, then dry-fry the onions and garlic over a high heat for 3–4 minutes, seasoning well with black pepper. Add the peppers and mushrooms and continue cooking for 1–2 minutes, then stir in the prawns, cabbage and the black bean and soy sauces and toss well.
2 Once the prawns have changed colour, add the remaining ingredients, toss well and heat through before serving.
3 For a dinner option, serve with 1 blue Portion Pot® (55g uncooked weight) or 1 red Portion Pot® (144g cooked weight) basmati rice per person.

Prawn Saag

SERVES 4
Per serving
118 calories 1.3g fat
Preparation 10 minutes
Cooking 20 minutes

175g cooked shelled prawns
1 red onion, finely chopped
2 garlic cloves, crushed
1 green pepper, deseeded and finely diced
1 × 400g can chopped tomatoes
300ml tomato passata
1 green chilli, seeded and finely chopped
200g fresh spinach
salt and freshly ground black pepper
chopped fresh coriander to garnish

1 Rinse the prawns well under cold running water.
2 Preheat a non-stick frying pan, then dry-fry the onion for 2–3 minutes until soft.
3 Add the garlic and green pepper to the pan and cook for 2–3 minutes. Stir in the tomatoes, tomato passata and chilli, and bring the sauce to a gentle simmer, then add the prawns and the spinach and heat through.
4 Season to taste with salt and black pepper before serving and garnish with the coriander.
5 For a dinner option, serve with 1 green Portion Pot® (170g) cooked egg noodles or 1 blue Portion Pot® (55g uncooked weight) or 1 red Portion Pot® (144g cooked weight) basmati rice per person.

TIP This sauce also works well with chicken or, for a vegetarian version, you can substitute Quorn pieces

Singapore Noodles with Prawns

SERVES 4
Per serving
212 calories 3.4g fat
Preparation 10 minutes
Cooking 20 minutes

110g fine noodles
2 leeks, finely sliced
2 garlic cloves, crushed
1 red pepper, deseeded and finely sliced
1 × 5cm piece lemongrass, finely chopped
175g mangetout
3 tbsps pineapple juice
1 tbsp soy sauce
225g peeled uncooked prawns
225g beansprouts
salt and freshly ground black pepper

1 Cook the noodles in boiling water, then drain.
2 Preheat a non-stick wok, then dry-fry the leeks and garlic until soft. Add the red pepper, lemongrass, mangetout, pineapple juice and soy sauce and toss well together. Stir in the prawns and cook until they change colour. Stir in the beansprouts and drained noodles and combine well. Serve hot.
3 For a lunch option, serve with a crisp salad.

TIP For a vegetarian option, use Quorn pieces instead of prawns

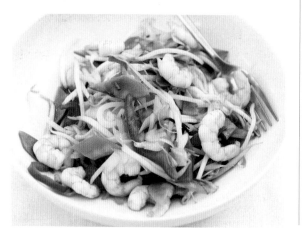

VEGETARIAN

Leek and Sage Meatballs ☑ with Pasta

SERVES 4
Per serving
390 calories 7.7g fat
Preparation 10 minutes
Cooking 25 minutes

500g Quorn mince
2 leeks, finely chopped
1 garlic clove, crushed
1 tbsp finely chopped sage
1 tbsp grainy mustard
1 tsp vegetable stock powder
1 egg, beaten
500g tomato passata
1 tbsp chopped fresh basil, plus extra for the garnish
1 tsp runny honey
200g (dry weight) pasta shapes
freshly ground black pepper
10g low-fat mature cheese to serve

1 Place the Quorn mince in a mixing bowl. Add the leeks, garlic, sage, mustard and stock powder and mix well. Mix in the beaten egg, then divide the mixture into 20 golfball-sized balls.
2 Preheat a non-stick pan, then dry-fry the meatballs, browning them on all sides. Add the tomato passata, 1 tbsp of basil and the honey and season with black pepper.
3 Meanwhile, cook the pasta in a pan of boiling water, then drain well and transfer to warmed serving bowls.
4 Spoon the sauce on top and garnish with the remaining basil and a little grated low-fat mature cheese.

TIP As a variation you can substitute beef, chicken or pork mince for the Quorn

Garlic Mushroom Pasta ☑

SERVES 4
Per serving
270 calories 4.5g fat
Preparation 10 minutes
Cooking 20 minutes

200g (dry weight) pasta shapes
1 vegetable stock cube
3 baby leeks (240g total), finely sliced
2 garlic cloves, crushed
200g button mushrooms
a few chilli flakes
200g Philadelphia Extra Light soft cheese
100ml semi-skimmed milk
1 tbsp chopped fresh basil
salt and freshly ground black pepper
olive oil spray

1 Cook the pasta in a pan of water containing the
   stock cube.
2 Preheat a non-stick pan, then dry-fry the leeks,
   garlic and mushrooms for 2–3 minutes in a little
   olive oil spray, taking care not to burn the garlic.
3 Add the chilli flakes and cheese, then season with
   salt and black pepper and cook for 8–10 minutes,
   adding enough milk to make a coating sauce.
   Finally, stir in the coriander.
4 Drain the pasta well, return it to the pan, then add
   the sauce and toss well. Serve straight away with a
   small salad.

*TIP You can also serve this mushroom sauce
with warm pitta slices instead of pasta*

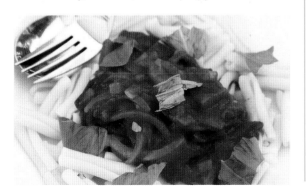

Roasted Pepper Pasta ☑

SERVES 4
Per serving
247 calories 1.5g fat
Preparation 20 minutes
Cooking 25 minutes

2 long red peppers (approx. 300g total)
200g (dry weight) pasta shapes
1 vegetable stock cube
1 red onion, finely sliced
2 garlic cloves, crushed,
1 × 500g pack tomato passata
salt and freshly ground black pepper
olive oil spray
chopped fresh basil to garnish

1 Preheat the oven to 200C, 400F, Gas Mark 6.
2 Put the peppers on a non-stick baking tray, spray
   lightly with olive oil and season with salt and
   pepper.
3 Place the peppers in the oven for 15–20 minutes
   until their skins start to lift away. Remove from the
   oven, cover the peppers completely with clear food
   wrap and leave to cool until the skins come away.
   Peel and chop the peppers and remove the seeds.
4 Cook the pasta in a large saucepan of boiling
   water with the stock cube.
5 Meanwhile, preheat a non-stick pan, then dry-fry
   the onion and garlic until soft. Add the peppers
   and passata and bring to a gentle simmer.
6 Drain the pasta thoroughly, arrange on warmed
   plates, pour the pepper sauce over and garnish
   with the basil.
7 Serve with a large salad tossed in fat-free dressing.

*TIP Add a pinch of dried chilli flakes to spice up
the sauce*

◀ *Roasted pepper pasta*

Quorn and Rice Bake ☑

SERVES 4
Per serving
339 calories 5g fat
Preparation 15 minutes
Cooking 25 minutes

2 medium red onions, cut into wedges
2 garlic cloves, crushed
2 celery sticks, chopped
1 red pepper, deseeded and diced
1 red chilli, sliced
4 Quorn fillets, cut into chunks
225g (dry weight) basmati rice
2 tsps vegetable stock powder
1 × 400g can chopped tomatoes
600ml water
salt and freshly ground black pepper
chopped fresh parsley to garnish

1 Preheat the oven 200C, 400F, Gas Mark 6. Preheat a non-stick frying pan.
2 Dry-fry the onions in the non-stick pan until lightly browned, then add the garlic, celery, pepper, chilli and Quorn. Stir in the rice, stock powder and tomatoes, and pour in sufficient water (approx. 600ml) to cover the rice. Bring to the boil, then reduce the heat and simmer gently for 20 minutes until the liquid has been absorbed and the rice is cooked.
3 Season to taste with black pepper before serving and garnish with the chopped parsley.
4 For a dinner option, serve with unlimited vegetables (excluding potatoes).

TIP Keep the vegetables quite chunky to add texture to the finished dish

Bombay Rice ☑❄

SERVES 4
Per serving
212 calories 2.1g fat
Preparation 10 minutes
Cooking 20 minutes

1 red onion, finely chopped
2 garlic cloves, crushed
1 red pepper, deseeded and diced
160g (dry weight) brown basmati rice
1 tbsp fajita mix powder
110g frozen peas
1 small red chilli, finely sliced
500ml vegetable stock
2 tbsps chopped fresh parsley
salt and freshly ground black pepper

1 Preheat a large non-stick pan, then dry-fry the onion, garlic and red pepper until soft.
2 Add the rice, fajita mix powder, peas and chilli, then pour in the stock and cook over a high heat until the rice is cooked and has absorbed all the liquid.
3 Just before serving sprinkle with the parsley. Serve with salad.

TIP For a main dish, add a few cooked vegetables or stir in some cooked prawns

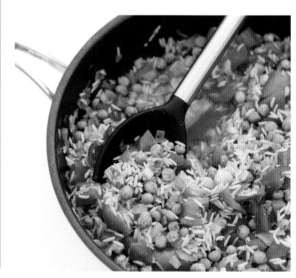

Stir-Fried Rice Noodles ☑

SERVES 1
Per serving
186 calories 1.4g fat
Preparation 10 minutes
Cooking 10 minutes

30g rice noodles
2 baby leeks, finely sliced 200g
½ garlic clove, crushed
½ yellow pepper, deseeded and sliced
2 baby courgettes, sliced
50g chestnut mushrooms, sliced
2 tsps soy sauce
1 tsp rice vinegar
squeeze of fresh lemon juice
freshly ground black pepper

1 Cook the rice noodles in boiling water and drain.
2 Preheat a non-stick wok, then add the leeks and garlic and dry-fry over a high heat for 3–4 minutes, seasoning well with black pepper. Add the yellow pepper, courgettes and mushrooms and continue cooking for 1–2 minutes. Stir in the cooked noodles along with the remaining ingredients and toss well together. Serve straight away.

TIP For a fresh herb flavour, add some chopped coriander to the noodles as you drain them

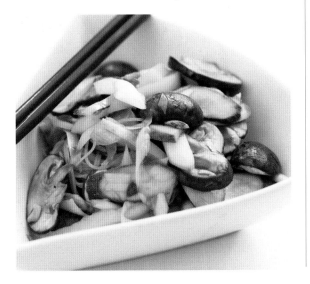

Cauliflower Bhaji ☑

SERVES 4
Per serving
107 calories 2.2g fat
Preparation 10 minutes
Cooking 20 minutes

2 red onions, chopped
2 garlic cloves, crushed
1 red pepper, deseeded and diced
1 cauliflower (300g), broken into florets
1 tbsp medium curry powder
2–3 curry leaves
1 green chilli, finely chopped
1 × 400g can chopped tomatoes
1–2 tsps vegetable stock powder
1 tbsp tomato purée
salt and freshly ground black pepper

1 Preheat a large non-stick pan, then dry-fry the onions and garlic for 1–2 minutes until soft. Add the red pepper, cauliflower and curry powder and cook for a further 5 minutes.
2 Stir in the remaining ingredients, add sufficient water to cook the cauliflower, and simmer gently for 10 minutes until the cauliflower is cooked, topping up with a little extra water if required.

TIP Serve this simple curry as a side dish with meat or fish or as a vegetarian main course with rice

Greek Salad Wrap ☑

MAKES 2
Per wrap
279 calories 6.6g fat
Preparation 5 minutes
Cooking 1–2 minutes

2 tortilla wraps
2 tbsps Philadelphia Extra Light soft cheese
4 fresh mint leaves, chopped
few rocket leaves
2 tomatoes, sliced
½ red pepper, deseeded and finely chopped
thinly sliced cucumber
freshly ground black pepper

1 Preheat a health grill or conventional grill to high.
2 Spread the tortillas with the cheese. Sprinkle the
   mint leaves over and add the rocket leaves,
   tomatoes, red pepper and cucumber, then season
   with black pepper. Roll up the tortillas, folding the
   ends in.
3 Place the wraps on the health grill or under the
   conventional grill for 1–2 minutes. Serve warm.

*TIP Pep up these wraps with some pickled
chillies*

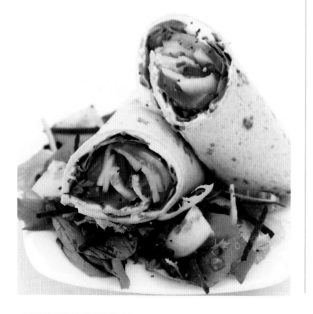

DESSERTS

Tropical Sorbet ❄

SERVES 8
Per serving
74 calories 0.1 g fat
Preparation 20 minutes
Cooking 10 minutes
Freezing 7 hours

110g caster sugar
1 ripe mango, peeled and sliced
2 passion fruit, seeds removed
1 papaya, peeled and seeds removed
zest and juice of 1 lemon
1 egg white

1 In a saucepan dissolve the sugar in 300ml water
   and bring to the boil, then remove from the heat
   and allow to cool.
2 Place all the fruit in a liquidiser and blend until
   smooth.
3 Mix the fruit with the cooled syrup, add the lemon
   zest and juice and pour into a shallow freezer
   container. Freeze for about 3 hours until mushy.
4 Whisk the egg white until stiff and fold into the
   loosened sorbet. Refreeze for 4 hours or overnight
   until firm.
5 Serve in chilled glasses with additional fruit if
   desired.

*TIP Remove the sorbet from the freezer 5
minutes before required to allow to it to soften
before serving*

Strawberry and Rhubarb Mousse

SERVES 6
Per serving
125 calories 2.9g fat
Preparation 20 minutes

1 × 410g can Carnation Light evaporated milk
340g fresh strawberries, hulled
6 sticks rhubarb (900g total), chopped
2 tbsps ginger wine or ginger ale
1 tbsp caster sugar
6 gelatine leaves
pinch of sugar
2 egg whites

1 Chill the Carnation milk overnight in the refrigerator or place in the freezer for 30 minutes until cold.
2 Using an electric whisk, whisk the milk until thick and creamy.
3 Reserve 4 strawberries and place the remainder in a saucepan. Add the rhubarb, ginger wine or ale and caster sugar and bring to the boil.
4 Soften the gelatine in cold water, then squeeze out the water, add the gelatine to the pan and stir well until dissolved.
5 Pour the fruit mixture into a blender and blend until smooth. If you wish, you can strain the mixture through a sieve to remove the seeds.
6 In a separate bowl, whisk the egg whites until stiff, adding a pinch of sugar. Fold the egg whites into the chilled, whisked milk, then fold in the raspberry purée.
7 Pour into serving glasses, decorate with the reserved strawberries and chill until ready to serve.

Strawberry and Rhubarb Mousse ▶

Coffee and Apricot Roulade

SERVES 8
Per serving
108 calories 0.2g fat
Preparation 5 minutes
Cooking 20 minutes

4 egg whites
175g caster sugar
2 tsps instant coffee granules
4 tbsps 0% fat Greek yogurt
3 fresh apricots, chopped

1 Preheat the oven to 150C, 300F, Gas Mark 2.
2 In a clean, dry bowl, whisk the egg whites to stiff peaks, then fold in the caster sugar a dessertspoon at a time, at 10-second intervals.
3 Pour the mixture onto a baking tray lined with baking parchment. Sprinkle the coffee granules over, then swirl the granules into the mixture.
4 Bake in the oven for 20 minutes, then remove the meringue from the oven, turn out onto foil and allow to cool.
5 When the meringue is cool, spread with the Greek yogurt, top with the apricots, then roll up lengthways to form a roulade.

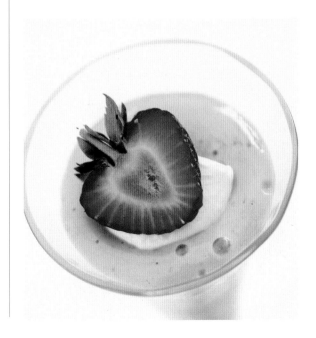

Banana Muffins

MAKES 6
Per muffin
99 calories 3.9g fat
Preparation 10 minutes
Cooking 20 minutes

3 tbsps Alpro cream alternative
1 tsp cider vinegar
2 tbsps golden caster sugar
1 × 100g banana
lemon juice
2 eggs, beaten
2 tbsps gluten-free flour
1 tsp gluten-free baking powder
1 tbsp icing sugar
speck of turmeric

1 Preheat the oven to 150C, 350F, Gas Mark 4.
2 Line a 6-hole muffin tin with papers. Whisk together the Alpro, vinegar and sugar until light and fluffy. Cut 6 thin slices from the banana (reserve the remainder) and place in a little lemon juice. Mash the remaining banana and add to the mix. Add the eggs, flour and baking powder, blending well together. Spoon into the papers and bake in the oven for 20 minutes.
3 Remove from oven and allow to cool. Mix together the icing sugar with the turmeric, add a little boiling water and stir until smooth. Pour onto the cakes and top with the reserved banana slices.

TIP Store these gluten-free muffins in an airtight container and keep for up to 2 days

Plum Tatin

SERVES 6
Per serving
107 calories 0.8g fat
Preparation 10 minutes
Cooking 30 minutes

6 dark plums
2 tbsps caster sugar
4 sheets filo pastry
low-calorie spray oil

1 Preheat the oven 200C, 400F, Gas Mark 6. Preheat a non-stick frying pan.
2 Remove the stones from the plums, place the stoned plums in the hot pan, add the sugar and cook over a low heat until the sugar starts to colour. Remove the plums from the pan and place in the base of a silicone cake mould.
3 Add 2 tbsps of water to the pan (be careful of the steam as the water comes into contact with the hot sugar). Heat until the sugar is dissolved, then pour over the plums. Layer the filo pastry sheets on top, spraying in between the layers with a little spray oil.
5 Bake in the oven for 15–20 minutes until golden in colour, then remove from the oven and allow to cool slightly before turning out onto a serving plate. Serve hot or cold with low-fat yogurt.

TIP Choose firm plums that will stand up to cooking – avoid over-ripe ones as they will become soft and lose their shape

Frozen Berry Smoothie

SERVES 1
Per serving
181 calories 0.7g fat
Preparation 5 minutes

50g frozen blueberries
50g frozen raspberries
1 small banana
200ml apple juice

1 Place all the ingredients into a smoothie maker or liquidiser and blend until smooth.
2 Serve as a speedy breakfast or dessert.

TIP If the mixture is too thick, add a little boiling water to thin it down

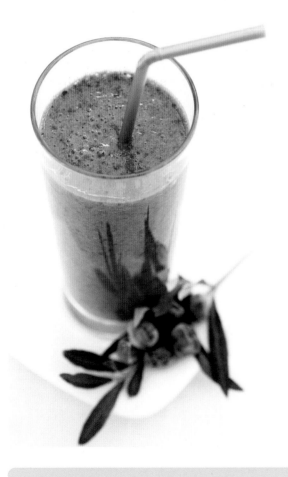

Crunchy Apple and Blackberry Pie

SERVES 4
Per serving
139 calories 0.8g fat
Preparation 15 minutes
Cooking 20 minutes

600g cooking apples
2 tsps salt
200g blackberries
2 tbsps golden caster sugar
2 sheets (100g total) filo pastry
pinch of mixed spice
low-calorie cooking oil spray

1 Preheat the oven to 150C, 300F, Gas Mark 2.
2 Peel and slice the apples into a bowl of salted water. Rinse well and place in the bottom of an ovenproof dish. Scatter the blackberries over and sprinkle with 1 tbsp of the sugar.
3 Cut the filo pastry sheets in half to give 4 sheets. Spray a sheet lightly with oil spray and place on top of the fruit, scrunching it up to give a wrinkled effect. Repeat with the other sheets, until the fruit is covered.
4 Spray the top sheet lightly with oil spray, sprinkle with the remaining sugar and dust with the mixed spice.
5 Bake in the centre of the oven for 20 minutes until crisp and golden. Serve hot or cold with low-fat yogurt.

TIP Slicing the apples into salted water and then rinsing them prevents them from turning brown as well as adding flavour

Maintaining your new weight

Once you have arrived at your ultimate goal weight, you'll want to maintain your new, slim figure and you may be worrying about what to do next.

Eating

To avoid weight gain, you need to continue with the low-fat, low-Gi, principles of eating. If you have found that eating more protein is helpful, then carry on with this. If you go back to eating high-fat snacks, cooking with fat and using fatty or oily dressings on your food, you will only pile back on the fat that you've worked so very hard to lose. Just as you can wean yourself away from the taste of high-fat foods, it is easy to retrain yourself back into your old, bad habits again and, if you do, you will regret it. This doesn't mean that you can't ever have a cream cake, a packet of crisps or a Big Mac. Of course you can. But only occasionally and it needs to be seen as a treat, and an exception rather than the rule.

You can increase your calories by a couple of hundred calories a day for the next three or four weeks. Then up the calories a little more and see if you are able to keep your weight constant. If you find the weight starts to creep back on, cut down again. Or if you have overindulged, for instance after a holiday or Christmas break, you can return to the 14-Day Fast Track diet, but unless your daily calorie allowance determines that that is the correct number of calories for your daily needs – which might be the case if you are aged 60 or over or have a small frame, or both – don't stick to it long term, as it could be counter-productive.

If you are aged 60 or over, you will not be able to eat more than about 1500 calories a day without putting on weight unless you do a lot of exercise. Hopefully, you will fall into a routine that allows you to eat enough and stay slim without feeling that you are dieting. Try to relax and gradually you will build your self-confidence in controlling your eating.

Exercise

Continue with 30 minutes of aerobic activity three to five times a week at a level that makes you mildly breathless and warm so that you achieve fat-burning mode. If you like working out to fitness DVDs, try my latest one, Rosemary Conley's Real Results Workout. It is a brilliant all-round programme and offers a 30-minute aerobic fat-burning workout, two 20-minute highly effective toning sections and two 'Express' workouts that take less than five minutes each. All my fitness DVDs give you a fabulous fat-burning whole body workout, but the main thing is that anyone can do them, as every move is demonstrated at different levels of ability to suit both the most fit and the least fit of followers.

If you want to continue with the exercises in this book, just repeat the exercises included in the last two weeks of the 28-day programme. Work at a level that challenges you so when you are able to increase the number of reps, do so, to reach a level where you can feel mild discomfort, and then do two more.

Once you have become fitter, and your muscles stronger and well toned, it doesn't take endless exercise to keep your body fit and trim. But if you don't use it, you will lose it!

The diet trial

Over the years I have held several trials to test my diets. It's helpful for me to have ordinary folk who lead regular lives follow my diets, because it provides real proof that the diet in question works and is 'followable'. Their comments, observations and experiences also enable me to tweak the diet to make it more practical and, therefore, more effective in the long term.

I had previously carried out two trials to determine how much weight could be lost safely in two weeks on an eating plan based on 1200 calories a day. With this Amazing Inch Loss Plan, I wanted to see if men and women alike could continue for a second two-week period on a relatively low number of calories in the hope of proving that a total weight loss of a stone could be achieved in four weeks. Prior to creating this strict four-week diet, I took professional advice from Dr Susan Jebb, a nutrition scientist, on whether it would be safe to ask men and women of any age and fitness to follow a two-week 1200-calorie diet followed by a two-week diet of 1400 calories. She confirmed it would be perfectly healthy for them to do so, providing they ate a well-balanced diet, took a multivitamin supplement and stayed properly hydrated, so I set about creating this two-stage plan.

Next, I appeared on BBC Radio Leicester to ask for volunteers to try the diet. Radio Leicester has helped me with trials before, even as far back as 1986 for my original Hip and Thigh Diet, and the listeners are really supportive. Radio presenter Tony Wadsworth is a great guy and his wife, Julie Mayer, who is a roving reporter for Radio Leicester, is a real fitness fan. During the four-week trial, she carried out several radio interviews with some of the slimmers, who described their progress on the diet. It made the whole experience great fun.

In selecting my volunteers I wanted people who, ideally, were 'virgin' dieters so that I could get as accurate a result as possible. 'Serial' dieters usually come with their own views of what works and what doesn't and would have been less likely to stick with the trial for the full four weeks. I also wanted my trial dieters to be committed to exercising almost every day. Serial dieters are notoriously not keen on exercise.

Fifty folk – both men and women – were chosen from the applications I received and their ages ranged from 18 to 70 years, with the average age being 48 years. Their weights ranged from 10st 5lb to 22st 1lb, and the average weight was 15st 6lb.

Each volunteer was given the option of following either the high protein or the high carbohydrate meal options and we ended up with 25 slimmers in each category. Interestingly, the average weight loss of each group was exactly the same – one stone in the four weeks of the trial!

The greatest weight loss in 28 days was seen by 63-year-old Bill Wiltshire, who shed an astonishing 1st 10lb – the most I have ever known anyone to lose in a month! Bill started off at 22st 1lb and, four weeks later, weighed in at 20st 5lb, plus he lost 23 inches in total from his body, including five inches from his waist.

Twenty-one year old Ryan Flack lost 1st 9lb, reducing his weight from 21st 12lb to 20st 3lb and his body fat percentage by almost five per cent – an extraordinary achievement in just four weeks.

Our top female slimmer on the trial was 18-year-old Jane Gillespie, who slimmed down from 11st 5lb to 9st 12lb and dropped two dress sizes in four weeks!

The trial dieters came to our head office at Quorn House each week to be weighed and measured by two members of my staff – Bridget Key, who used to be a franchisee for our Clubs but now works at head office as the Start-Up Manager for our new franchisees, and Sue White, whom I appointed as my researcher for the trial. The dieters were weighed on our special, and rather sophisticated, scales, which also measure body fat percentage. In addition to calculating each person's body mass index (BMI) and basal metabolic rate (BMR), these scales also predicted their 'metabolic age' based on all the information given and the readings taken.

When trial dieter Andy Corbett first weighed in, his metabolic age was calculated at 55 years – 10 years older than Andy's actual age of 45. After four weeks on the diet, Andy lost an amazing 1st 8lb (slimming from 15st 12lb to 14st 5lb), and his metabolic age reduced by 15 years, from 55 to 40!

Andy decided that he would rather exercise early in the day, so at six o'clock each morning he worked out to one of my DVDs. He told me that he and his wife had never laughed so much as he initially struggled with his co-ordination and felt his flab wobbling about as he exercised. After a month, he admitted that the workouts were no longer as entertaining and his wife didn't laugh as much because he could execute the routines much better now that his beer-belly and man-boobs had almost disappeared! Andy lost four inches from his waist in the four weeks.

Mark Clayton slimmed down from 16st 1lb to 14st 11lb, losing a total of 1st 4lb. Mark is 45 years old, but when he started the diet his predicted metabolic age was 60. After just four weeks his metabolic age had gone down to 38 years!

As we get older, our metabolic rate reduces, so I expected that my older trial dieters would not achieve anything like the average one-stone weight loss over the four weeks, but six out of the eleven over-60s did lose a stone or more.

The lowest weight loss achieved was 8lb and there were several people who lost 11, 12 and 13lb, which was still excellent, and they were delighted with their results. Deana Merry lost 12lb, even though she went on holiday to France during the trial. And Sue Vickers admitted that she hadn't stuck rigidly to the diet but nevertheless lost 8lb and 16¾ inches in four weeks.

On the final weighing in day, the atmosphere was electric. Everyone seemed so happy and all the members of the trial team looked notably slimmer. The room was buzzing with stories of how their doctors had reduced their blood pressure tablets or diabetes medication and how the pains in their knees, hips, ankles had diminished! They all felt so much healthier and couldn't believe how quickly they

had become accustomed to eating less than before and yet they hadn't gone hungry. They had enjoyed exercising and being part of the trial and were very grateful for the chance to improve their health. Dave Goodman, who lost 1st 5lb, explained to me that he'd had a fairly serious chest complaint but, after losing his excess weight, he hadn't had to use his inhaler for three weeks!

To top it all, the trial dieters had achieved an **average weight loss of 14lb** and lost an **average of 13.3 inches from their bodies in the four weeks**. I was thrilled and I felt confident that anyone else who followed the diet in this book, with all the motivational messages, daily exercises and menu suggestions at their fingertips, really could lose a stone in a month, and I was happy to make this claim.

Here are some additional comments from members of the trial team:

'This was my first diet and I can't believe how easy it was to follow and that I lost 1st 9lb in the first month! I am amazed!'
Ryan Flack (lost 1st 9lb)

'This is the easiest diet I have ever known. I can't believe the results after just four weeks. I don't feel so sleepy, my skin is much clearer and I feel much more confident. It has certainly changed my life and the way I think and feel about food. I am now well on the way to a new me!'
Helen McLeod (lost 10lb)

'My weight would not budge until I followed this diet. I don't feel I've been on a diet but a healthy eating plan that I plan to keep following. I feel so much better and can now wear clothes I had "grown out of"! Thank you!'
Gillian Betts (lost 1st)

'I really didn't believe I could eat so much food and lose weight, but it works. I don't want this good feeling to end! My health has improved, my self-esteem is returning, I feel feminine again. I actually went in to a shop and bought a new dress and it fitted! I was so excited.'
Susan Bishop (lost 13lb)

'Both me and my doctor are very happy! Losing so much weight in just a month, and so easily, is amazing!'
Bill Wiltshire (lost 1st 10lb)

'I have enjoyed this diet and have never achieved such a good result on any other diet.'
Louise Slingsby (lost 1st)

'I have completely lost my beer belly and man boobs. Brilliant! I have really enjoyed the trial. I work out to the DVD every morning for 30 minutes. My wife says I've lost my stomach and I've stopped snoring at night. I sleep better, feel better and am generally much happier. My get up and go has come back and I feel so fit! The other morning I was walking around a park and I hadn't noticed my shorts were falling down, showing my summer-patterned underpants. This is the fashion for teenagers, not a 45-year-old!'
Andy Corbett (lost 1st 6lb)

'Thank you for letting me be one of the lucky ones. I really enjoyed doing the trial and will be carrying on doing it now my mind is in the zone and I have seen such great results. The diet was easy to follow and I didn't miss anything really.'
Polly Gray (lost 10lb)

'I lost almost a stone in four weeks, but the biggest shock was my inch loss! I no longer suffer from heartburn or acid indigestion. I have more energy and can walk without getting out of breath. I can't believe how much food you can eat in one day!'
Jeanette Hopkins (lost 13½lb)

'This was my first ever diet and I am amazed at the results. It is so easy to follow, tasted great and I didn't feel I was missing out. I am really pleased that my cholesterol has also significantly reduced.'
Mark Clayton (lost 1st 4lb)

'I feel so much healthier, and my confidence has gone sky high! My hubby thinks I'm up to no good because I'm wearing nice clothes and looking in the mirror more!'
Deana Merry (lost 12lb)

'Wow! I was absolutely thrilled. I lost 16¾ inches in total in only four weeks – including four inches from my waist. Thank you! It has really made a difference to my life.'
Sue Vickers (lost 8lb)

'Great diet. Really simple and effective and it retrained your brain and stomach to eat much smaller portions without you even realising it. And it works!'
Teresa O'Neill (lost 11lb)

'Before this diet I was under the illusion that, because of my age [60], it would be almost impossible to lose any weight. You have proved me wrong. Thank you!'
Leslie Charles (lost 10lb)

'I felt such jubilation at losing a stone. Now I need to move forward and lose more – the best of the rest of my life is just around the corner!'
Julie Neville (lost 1st 1lb)

Your personal calorie allowance (women)

Check against your current weight and age range to find the ideal daily calorie allowance that will give you a healthy rate of weight loss after you've completed the initial 28-day plan.

Women aged 18–29			Women aged 30–59			Women aged 60–74		
Body Weight		(BMR)	Body Weight		(BMR)	Body Weight		(BMR)
Stones	Kilos	Calories	Stones	Kilos	Calories	Stones	Kilos	Calories
7	45	1147	7	45	1208	7	45	1048
7.5	48	1194	7.5	48	1233	7.5	48	1073
8	51	1241	8	51	1259	8	51	1099
8.5	54	1288	8.5	54	1285	8.5	54	1125
9	57	1335	9	57	1311	9	57	1151
9.5	60.5	1382	9.5	60.5	1337	9.5	60.5	1176
10	64	1430	10	64	1373	10	64	1202
10.5	67	1477	10.5	67	1389	10.5	67	1228
11	70	1524	11	70	1414	11	70	1254
11.5	73	1571	11.5	73	1440	11.5	73	1279
12	76	1618	12	76	1466	12	76	1305
12.5	80	1665	12.5	80	1492	12.5	80	1331
13	83	1712	13	83	1518	13	83	1357
13.5	86	1760	13.5	86	1544	13.5	86	1382
14	89	1807	14	89	1570	14	89	1408
14.5	92	1854	14.5	92	1595	14.5	92	1434
15	95.5	1901	15	95.5	1621	15	95.5	1460
15.5	99	1948	15.5	99	1647	15.5	99	1485
16	102	1995	16	102	1673	16	102	1511
16.5	105	2043	16.5	105	1699	16.5	105	1537
17	108	2090	17	108	1725	17	108	1563
17.5	111	2137	17.5	111	1751	17.5	111	1588
18	115	2184	18	115	1776	18	115	1614
18.5	118	2231	18.5	118	1802	18.5	118	1640
19	121	2278	19	121	1828	19	121	1666
19.5	124	2325	19.5	124	1854	19.5	124	1691
20	127	2373	20	127	1880	20	127	1717

Your personal calorie allowance (men)

Check against your current weight and age range to find the ideal daily calorie allowance that will give you a healthy rate of weight loss after you've completed the initial 28-day plan.

Men aged 18–29				Men aged 30–59				Men aged 60–74		
Body Weight		(BMR)		Body Weight		(BMR)		Body Weight		(BMR)
Stones	Kilos	Calories		Stones	Kilos	Calories		Stones	Kilos	Calories
7	45	1363		7	45	1384		7	45	1232
7.5	48	1411		7.5	48	1421		7.5	48	1270
8	51	1459		8	51	1457		8	51	1307
8.5	54	1507		8.5	54	1494		8.5	54	1345
9	57	1555		9	57	1530		9	57	1383
9.5	60.5	1602		9.5	60.5	1567		9.5	60.5	1421
10	64	1650		10	64	1603		10	64	1459
10.5	67	1698		10.5	67	1640		10.5	67	1497
11	70	1746		11	70	1676		11	70	1535
11.5	73	1794		11.5	73	1713		11.5	73	1573
12	76	1842		12	76	1749		12	76	1611
12.5	80	1890		12.5	80	1786		12.5	80	1649
13	83	1938		13	83	1822		13	83	1687
13.5	86	1986		13.5	86	1859		13.5	86	1725
14	89	2034		14	89	1895		14	89	1763
14.5	92	2082		14.5	92	1932		14.5	92	1801
15	95.5	2129		15	95.5	1968		15	95.5	1839
15.5	99	2177		15.5	99	2005		15.5	99	1877
16	102	2225		16	102	2041		16	102	1915
16.5	105	2273		16.5	105	2078		16.5	105	1953
17	108	2321		17	108	2114		17	108	1991
17.5	111	2369		17.5	111	2151		17.5	111	2028
18	115	2417		18	115	2187		18	115	2066
18.5	118	2465		18.5	118	2224		18.5	118	2104
19	121	2513		19	121	2260		19	121	2142
19.5	124	2561		19.5	124	2297		19.5	124	2180
20	127	2609		20	127	2333		20	127	2218

Index of recipes

apples
    crunchy apple and blackberry pie
        225
apricots
    coffee and apricot roulade 223

bacon
    BLT bruschetta 198
    brunch pitta 216
baked liver and onions 202
bananas
    banana muffins 224
    frozen berry smoothie 225
barbecued garlic chicken 212
beef
    beef fajitas 201
    beef kebabs 201
    cheesy cottage pie 214
    pasta bolognese 202
    steak in mushroom sauce 202
bhaji, cauliflower 221
black bean prawns 217
blackberries
    crunchy apple and blackberry pie
        225
blueberries
    frozen berry smoothie 225
bolognese
    pasta bolognese 202
    quorn bolognese 203
bombay rice 220
broccoli and leek soup 210
brunch pitta 216

cauliflower bhaji 221
cheesy cottage pie 214
cheesy quorn bake 204
chicken
    barbecued garlic chicken 212
    chicken, mushroom and lemon soup
        210
    chicken in mushroom sauce 201
    chicken noodle soup 211
    chicken pasta 200
    chicken or quorn stir-fry 199
    chicken and rice salad 200
    chicken shaslik 212

chicken with couscous 201
chinese chicken kebabs 211
quick and easy chicken curry 201
salad bowl with prawns, chicken or
    ham 198
spicy chicken pasta 201
stir-fried chicken 199
stir-fry chicken with ginger 201
tuna or chicken pasta salad 200
chickpeas
    mixed bean salad 199
chilli prawn or quorn stir-fry with
    asparagus 122
chilli prawn stir-fry with peppers and
    mushrooms 203
chinese chicken kebabs 211
crunchy apple and blackberry pie 225
cod
    fish pie 203
coffee and apricot roulade 223
cottage pie, cheesy 214
couscous, with chicken 201
curry
    chicken shaslik 212
    quick and easy chicken curry 201

desserts
    banana muffins 224
    coffee and apricot roulade 223
    crunchy apple and blackberry pie
        225
    eton mess 206
    frozen berry smoothie 225
    fruit smoothie 196
    plum tatin 224
    strawberry and rhubarb mousse 223
    tropical sorbet 222

fish and seafood
    black bean prawns 217
    chilli prawn stir-fry with asparagus
        203
    chilli prawn stir-fry with peppers and
        mushrooms 203
    fish pie 203
    oven-baked salmon 203
    prawn saag 217

prawn wrap 198
salad bowl with prawns, chicken or
    ham 198
singapore noodles with prawns
    218
smoked salmon pasta salad 200
tuna or chicken pasta salad 200
frozen berry smoothie 225
fruit smoothie 196

gammon and liver kebabs 199
garlic mushroom pasta 219
goulash, lamb and mushroom 215
greek salad wrap 222

ham
    ham, leek and sweet potato pie
        216
    ham and cheese omelette 202
    salad bowl with prawns, chicken or
        ham 198
homemade vegetable soup 200

kebabs
    beef kebabs 201
    chinese chicken kebabs 211
    gammon and liver kebabs 199
kidney beans
    mixed bean salad 199
lamb
    lamb medallions with blackcurrant
        sauce 214
    lamb and mushroom goulash 215
    lamb stir-fry 202
leeks
    broccoli and leek soup 210
    ham, leek and sweet potato pie 216
    leek and sage meatballs with pasta
        218
liver
    baked liver and onions 202
    gammon and liver kebabs 199

mango
    tropical sorbet 222
meatballs, leek and sage, with pasta
    218

meringue
    coffee and apricot roulade 223
mixed bean salad 199
mixed grill 201
mousse, strawberry and rhubarb 223
muffins, banana 224
mushrooms
    chicken, mushroom and lemon soup 210
    chicken in mushroom sauce 201
    chilli prawn stir-fry with peppers and mushrooms 203
    garlic mushroom pasta 219
    lamb and mushroom goulash 215
    steak in mushroom sauce 202
    tomatoes and mushrooms on toast 197
noodles
    singapore noodles with prawns 218
    stir-fried rice noodles 221

omelette
    ham and cheese omelette 202
    spanish omelette 199
oven-baked salmon 203

passion fruit
    tropical sorbet 222
pasta
    chicken pasta 200
    garlic mushroom pasta 219
    leek and sage meatballs with pasta 218
    pasta bolognese 202
    pasta ratatouille 203
    quorn bolognese 203
    roasted pepper pasta 219
    smoked salmon pasta salad 200
    spicy chicken pasta 201
    tuna or chicken pasta salad 200
pitta, brunch 216
plum tatin 224
pork
    spicy pork steak 202
    sweet and sour pork chop 202
    wine braised pork slices 215
prawns
    black bean prawns 217
    chilli prawn stir-fry with asparagus 203
    chilli prawn stir-fry with peppers and mushrooms 203
    fish pie 203
    prawn saag 217

prawn wrap 198
    salad bowl with prawns, chicken or ham 198
    singapore noodles with prawns 218

quick and easy chicken curry 201
quorn
    cheesy quorn bake 204
    chilli quorn stir-fry with asparagus 204
    pasta bolognese 22
    quorn and rice bake 220
    sweet and sour quorn 204

raspberries
    frozen berry smoothie 225
ratatouille, pasta 203
rhubarb
    strawberry and rhubarb mousse 223
rice
    bombay rice 220
    chicken and rice salad 200
    quorn and rice bake 220
    stir-fried rice noodles 221
roasted pepper pasta 219
roulade
    coffee and apricot roulade 223

salads
    chicken and rice salad 200
    mixed bean salad 199
    salad bowl with prawns, chicken or ham 198
    smoked salmon pasta salad 200
    tuna or chicken pasta salad 200
salmon
    fish pie 203
    oven-baked salmon 203
    smoked salmon pasta salad 200
samosas, turkey and mango 213
singapore noodles with prawns 218
smoked salmon pasta salad 200
smoothie
    frozen berry smoothie 225
    fruit smoothie 196
sorbet, tropical 222
soups
    broccoli and leek 210
    chicken, mushroom and lemon 210
    chicken noodle 211
    homemade vegetable 200
southern fried turkey 213
spanish omelette 199
spicy chicken pasta 201

spicy pork steak 202
steak in mushroom sauce 202
stir-fries
    chilli prawn stir-fry with asparagus 203
    chilli prawn stir-fry with peppers and mushrooms 203
    stir-fried chicken 199
    stir-fried rice noodles 221
    stir-fry chicken with ginger 201
strawberries
    frozen berry smoothie 225
    strawberry and rhubarb mousse 223
sweet potato
    ham, leek and sweet potato pie 216
sweet and sour pork chop 202
sweet and sour quorn 204

tomatoes and mushrooms on toast 197
tropical sorbet 222
tuna or chicken pasta salad 200
turkey
    mixed grill 201
    southern fried turkey 213
    turkey and mango samosas 213

vegetarian
    bombay rice 220
    broccoli and leek soup 210
    cauliflower bhaji 221
    cheesy quorn bake 204
    chilli quorn stir-fry with asparagus 204
    garlic mushroom pasta 219
    greek salad wrap 222
    homemade vegetable soup 200
    leek and sage meatballs with pasta 218
    mixed bean salad 199
    pasta ratatouille 203
    quorn bolognese 203
    quorn and rice bake 220
    roasted pepper pasta 219
    spanish omelette 199
    stir-fried rice noodles 221
    sweet and sour quorn 146
    vegetable chilli 203

wine braised pork slices 215
wraps
    greek salad wrap 222
    prawn wrap 198

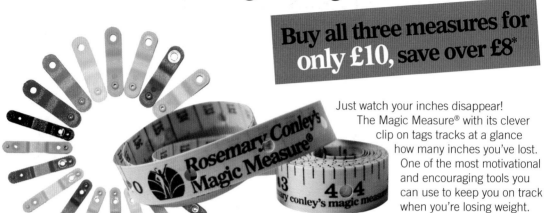
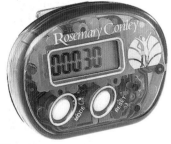
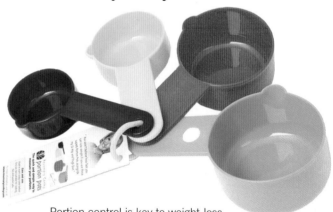

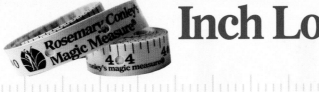
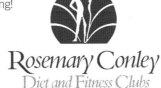
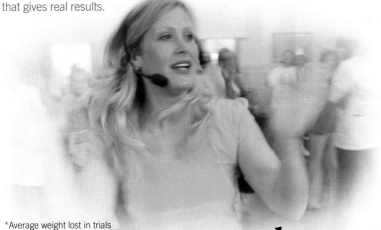
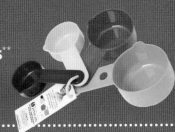

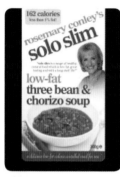
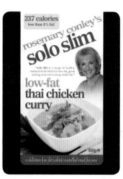
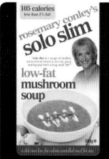
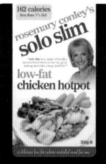
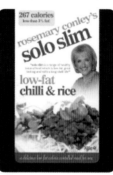
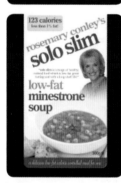
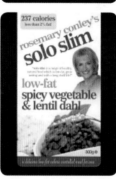
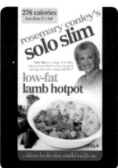
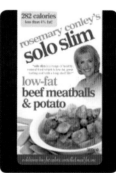

Lose a stone in a month *

with *Rosemary Conley's NEW* Amazing
Inch Loss Plan

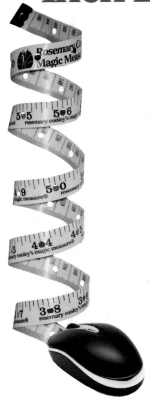

Turn on to www.rosemaryconleyonline.com
and turn off those cravings
Real inch loss results are just a click away

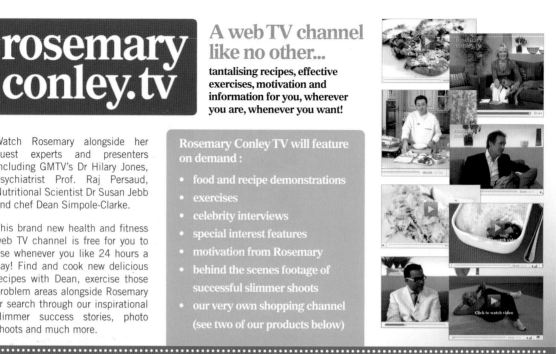
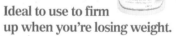
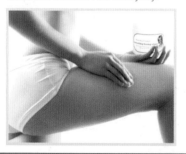

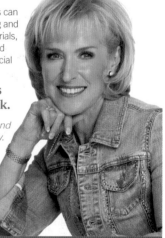

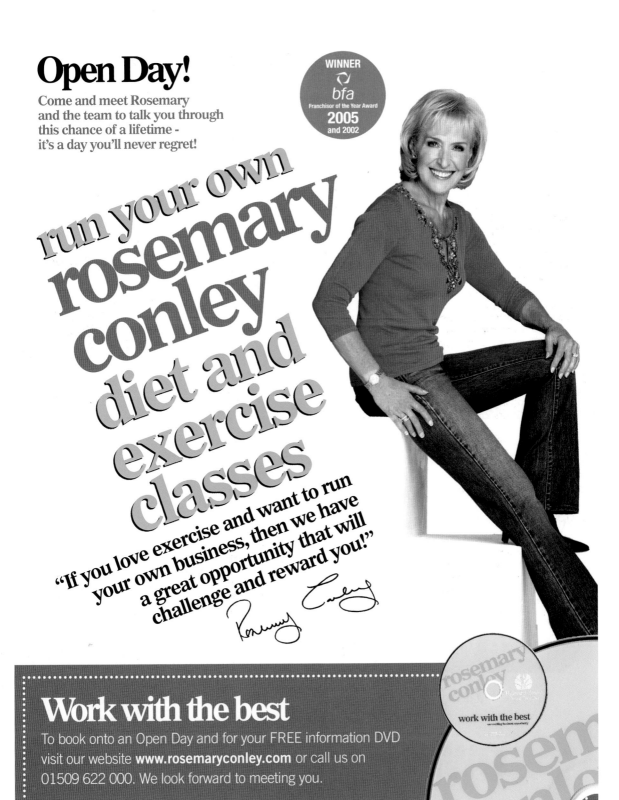

Open Day!

Come and meet Rosemary
and the team to talk you through
this chance of a lifetime -
it's a day you'll never regret!

WINNER
bfa
Franchisor of the Year Award
2005
and 2002

run your own
**rosemary
conley**
diet and
exercise
classes

"If you love exercise and want to run
your own business, then we have
a great opportunity that will
challenge and reward you!"

Achieve real results with Rosemary's last ever fitness DVD!

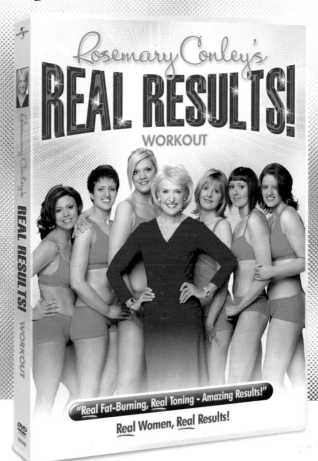

Lose weight, burn fat and tone up!

Each section is highly effective and always offers an easy or an advanced option. Whether you are new to exercise or really fit, this exercise programme will work for you.

OWN IT NOW ON DVD!